Diagnosis and Management of Alzheimer's Disease and Other Dementias

Second Edition

Robert C. Green, MD, MPH

Professor of Neurology,
Medicine (Genetics), and Epidemiology
Boston University Schools of
Medicine and Public Health

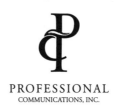

PROFESSIONAL
COMMUNICATIONS, INC.

Professional Communications, Inc.

A Medical Publishing Company

Marketing Office:
400 Center Bay Drive
West Islip, NY 11795
(t) 631/661-2852
(f) 631/661-2167

Editorial Office:
PO Box 10
Caddo, OK 74729-0010
(t) 580/367-9838
(f) 580/367-9989

For orders only, please call
1-800-337-9838
or visit our website at
www.pcibooks.com

ISBN: 1-884735-96-7

Printed in the United States of America

DISCLAIMER

The opinions expressed in this publication reflect those of the author. However, the author makes no warranty regarding the contents of the publication. The protocols described herein are general and may not apply to a specific patient. Any product mentioned in this publication should be taken in accordance with the prescribing information provided by the manufacturer.

This text is printed on recycled paper.

DEDICATION

This manual is dedicated to my patients and their caregivers who demonstrate enormous courage and inspiring dignity in the face of devastating illness; and to my teachers, colleagues, and students who struggle with them. I have taken particular inspiration from Joan Harrison, RN, GNP, and Eric Steinberg, MSN, RN, CS, and their dedication to the patients and families we have cared for together.

ACKNOWLEDGMENT

The author has been supported during the writing of this manual by grants from the National Institute on Aging and the National Human Genome Research Institute of the National Institutes of Health (P30 AG13846, RO1 AG09029, RO1 HG/AG02213, and U01 AG10483), as well as grants from the Alzheimer's Association.

In recent years, I have received funds for consultation or educational presentations from Eisai Pharma, Inc, Forest Pharmaceuticals, Inc, Janssen Pharmaceutica Products, LP, Novartis Pharmaceuticals Corporation, and Pfizer, Inc.

ABOUT THE AUTHOR

Dr. Green graduated from Amherst College and the University of Virginia School of Medicine before completing a residency in neurology at Harvard Medical School's Longwood Neurology Program. Following this, he completed research fellowships in Behavioral Neurology and Neurophysiology at the Beth Israel Hospital and Children's Hospital in Boston, where he was awarded both the William B. Lennox Research Fellowship and the Wilder Penfield Research Fellowship.

In 1988, Dr. Green joined the Department of Neurology at Emory University School of Medicine in Atlanta, Georgia, where he founded the Emory Neurobehavioral Program and Memory Assessment Clinics. He was appointed Chief of Neurology at Wesley Woods Geriatric Center and was the Clinical Director of Emory's Alzheimer's Disease Center. In Atlanta, Dr. Green obtained additional training in epidemiology, receiving a master's degree from the Rollins School of Public Health at Emory University.

In 1999, Dr. Green joined the faculty of Boston University School of Medicine, where he directs the Alzheimer's Disease Clinical and Research Program at Boston University School of Medicine. He is the author of over 120 publications, serves on a number of advisory, editorial, and grant review boards, and is past President of the Society for Behavioral and Cognitive Neurology. He has been voted one of America's "Best Doctors" by his peers.

Dr. Green's research interests are in early and preclinical detection, treatment, and prevention of Alzheimer's disease. He is the Associate Director and Clinical Core Director of Boston University's NIH-funded Alzheimer's Disease Center, co-Principal Investigator on Boston University's NIH-funded MIRAGE Study (Multi-Institutional Research in Alzheimer's Genetic Epidemiology), a consultant on the NIH-funded Cache County Memory and Aging Study, and Boston site director of the NIH-funded ADAPT Study (Alzheimer's Disease Anti-inflammatory Prevention Trial), one of the first large-scale intervention trials to prevent the development of Alzheimer's disease in at-risk family members. Dr. Green is also Principal Investigator and Director of the REVEAL Study (Risk Evaluation and Education for Alzheimer's disease), a new multicenter project (funded by the National Human Genome Research Institute and the National Institute on Aging) to develop genetic risk assessment strategies for individuals at risk for Alzheimer's disease.

For more information on these research studies, call toll-free 1-888-458-BUAD (2823) or see www.bualzresearch.org on the internet.

TABLE OF CONTENTS

TABLES

FIGURES

COLOR PLATES

Introduction

A dramatic demographic change is occurring in all developed countries, wherein the oldest segments of the population are increasing at the fastest rate. The population aged 65 and over is expected to increase from 33.5 million in 1995 to 39.4 million in 2010 and to over 69 million by 2030;[1] with these increases will come a virtual epidemic of age-related diseases. Some of the most frightening of these diseases are the progressive dementing disorders in which the very substance of life's experiences—our ability to make memories, to communicate with our families and friends, or even to maintain the essence of our identity—are lost.

The most common of the dementing disorders is Alzheimer's disease (AD), and recent years have brought unprecedented progress in understanding the genetics, pathophysiology, and natural history of this disease. The clinical care of patients with AD is still in its infancy but is rapidly evolving, with important new advances in diagnosis and pharmacologic and nonpharmacologic management. There are genetic and biochemical markers that may help with diagnosis and new pharmaceutical treatments that, for the first time, can improve both the cognitive and behavioral symptoms of the disease.

Of equal importance, there is a new understanding of the importance of patient and caregiver counseling, environmental and behavioral modification strategies, the value of social and legal planning, and the need to work with the entire family as "the patient."

This manual is designed for the neurologists, psychiatrists, and primary-care clinicians who are increasingly responsible for the diagnosis and management of the majority of dementing illnesses. It provides brief background sections describing the epidemiology and differential diagnosis of the dementing disorders. A section on AD highlights risk factors, biomarkers, and other diagnostic considerations, then concentrates on the natural history, pathophysiology, and current and emerging treatments for cognitive symptoms of AD. Specific attention is directed toward the evidence available on behalf of currently marketed biologic markers and pharmacologic therapies.

Additional chapters address topics common to most dementing illnesses, such as management of agitation, family and social/legal issues, and a listing of information and service resources, including web sites, that provide responsible information. In the final section of Chapter 11, *Resources for Clinicians and Families*, blanks have been left so that the primary-care clinician can fill in the phone numbers of local resource providers for easy reference.

1 Definitions of Dementia

Dementia as a Syndrome

Dementia is an acquired syndrome in which impairment of cognitive abilities is severe enough to interfere with the individual's customary occupational and social activities.[2,3] As conventionally used, dementia implies "degenerative" and "progressive," but it is also sometimes used in the context of static conditions (such as the cognitive impairment following stroke) or reversible conditions (such as cognitive impairment associated with overmedication or depression). Thus the term "dementia" is useful to communicate the presence of a syndrome but should not be used as a synonym for any particular diagnostic category, such as Alzheimer's disease (AD).

Dementia as Shorthand for Unsuccessful Aging

Dementia is often used to signal cognitive impairments that are considered abnormal for the age of the individual. For example, in a study of 40 American centenarians, only 23 met the author's criteria for dementia while 32 scored lower than 15 (an unequivocally impaired score) on the Mini-Mental State Examination.[4] In a similar study of 179 Finnish centenarians, 72 were considered to be demented by the author while 134 were considered to be cognitively impaired.[5,6] Obviously, some age-related handicap is being assumed in these reports, with the concept of dementia being loosely reserved for those persons whose symptoms are simply more severe or who are more functionally impaired than the author's expectations.

The struggle to ascertain what is normal about cognitive aging has an extensive literature and a long history of clinical ambivalence about the significance of mild memory impairments. The terms "benign senescent forgetfulness" and "age-associated memory impairment" have been used to emphasize the notion that such impairments were an inevitable nonpathologic concomitant of aging, at least in some patients. These terms should no longer be used at all because they were never well defined or validated through clinico-pathologic correlations. A more recent and constructive concept is mild cognitive impairment, used to describe older adults with mild memory deficits who are intact in other areas of cognition[7] and who are at increased risk for AD (see Chapter 6, *Natural History*).

Still, in many current publications and discussions, the term dementia is used to signal to the reader that the severity of the cognitive impairment exceeds what the writer expects to find in a person of that age. This shorthand is not useful since expectations are so variable, particularly among the oldest old.

Dementia as a Diagnosis

A long-standing area of confusion was clarified in the *Diagnostic and Statistical Manual of Mental Disorders*, fourth edition (DSM-IV).[8] Prior to this edition, the term dementia was an official diagnostic and billable diagnosis that did not clearly distinguish among etiologies, although the criteria described most closely resembled clinical criteria for AD. Many research studies have used DSM criteria for dementia, further compounding the confusion by setting precedents for the use of this term as a diagnostic entity in clinical research.

The authors of the DSM-IV have partially clarified this confusion in their latest version by defining dementia as a general diagnosis that requires a specific etiology. Nonetheless, the damage has been done, and the use of the term as a freestanding diagnostic label has an ineradicable pedigree.

Defining Dementia in the 21st Century

In light of these definitional issues, use of the term dementia should be clearly defined as a *syndrome of persistent cognitive impairment in adults*. The recognition of this syndrome should trigger an evaluation in every case in order to discover the cause(s) of symptoms and provide for diagnosis, treatment, and if necessary, long-term management of the patient.

2   Epidemiology of Dementia

As described in Chapter 1, *Definitions of Dementia*, in common usage, dementia is a broad term that may include many specific disorders. Therefore, a number of clinical definitions of dementia or of Alzheimer's disease (AD) have been used for case ascertainment in epidemiologic studies. Most of these studies have estimated *prevalence* (ie, the proportion of cases at a particular time), although some have estimated *incidence* (ie, the proportion of new cases arising over a specific period of time). Typically, epidemiologic studies of dementia utilize cases that are already diagnosed or they assess large numbers of subjects using relatively nonspecific testing. Studies that address the issue of relative frequency of different etiologies of dementia must use more elaborate diagnostic procedures. Using epidemiologic methods, numerous case-control (retrospective) studies and fewer cohort (prospective) studies have been carried out in order to look for environmental or genetic factors that may be more or less strongly associated with the syndrome of dementia or with AD.[9,10]

Prevalence of Dementia

Epidemiologic studies consistently indicate that prevalence of dementia doubles every 5 years between the ages of 65 and 85 (**Figure 2.1**).[11-26] As reflected in the broad tail of **Figure 2.1**, there is only a partial consensus about the prevalence of dementia among those who live beyond the age of 85. Several large population-based studies indicate that dementia prevalence remains high after the age of 85 and probably rises fur-

15

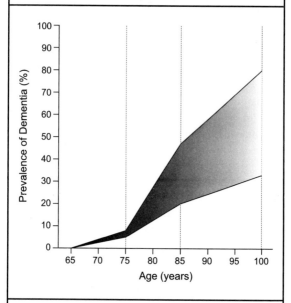

FIGURE 2.1 — ESTIMATES OF DEMENTIA PREVALENCE IN DIFFERENT AGE GROUPS

There is relative agreement about the prevalence of dementia in the sixth and seventh decades, but as this figure illustrates, there are diverging estimates of the prevalence of dementia among the oldest old.

Based on data from: Katzman R, Kawas C. In: *Alzheimer Disease*. 1994:105-122; O'Connor DW, et al. *Acta Psychiatr Scand*. 1989;79:190-198; Evans DA, et al. *JAMA*. 1989; 262:2551-2556; Heeren TJ, et al. *J Am Geriatr Soc*. 1991;39: 755-759; Aronson MK, et al. *Arch Intern Med*. 1991;151:989-992; Skoog I, et al. *N Engl J Med*. 1993;328:153-158; Ebly EM, et al. *Neurology*. 1994;44:1593-1600; Wernicke TF. *Neurology*. 1994;44:250-253; Johansson B, Zarit SH. *Int J Geriatr Psychiatry*. 1995;10:359-366; Ankri J, Poupard M. *Rev Epidemiol Sante Publique*. 2003;51:349-360.

ther with increasing age. However, based upon a relatively small number of persons over 90 years of age, some studies have suggested that the prevalence of dementia plateaus or even drops in the very old.[27-30] It has been estimated that by the year 2050, there will be over 13 million persons with dementia in the US population[31] and over 114 million persons with dementia worldwide.[32]

Incidence Rates of Dementia

Incidence studies of dementia are more difficult to do, because one must follow relatively large numbers of individuals over years. Like prevalence, incidence of dementia is thought to double approximately every few years, rising to rates of 2% to 6% after age 80.[12,33-35] Incidence rates in nonindustrialized countries are more difficult to ascertain because of misclassifications in those with lower education and lesser availability of diagnostic procedures such as CT or MR scans, but incidence appears to be similar to the United States in Spanish populations,[36] lower than expected among Yoruba residents of Nigeria,[37] and higher than expected among Arabs in the Wadi Ara region of Israel.[38] There is some evidence that incidence of AD declines in the ninth decade.[39] Efforts are underway to standardize the diagnosis of dementia in a large number of countries.[40]

Etiologies of Dementia

Some population-based studies have found nearly equal proportions of AD and vascular dementia, while others reveal a higher incidence of vascular dementia.[12,13,15,23,41] In the methodologically rigorous East Boston Study, a large majority of both prevalent and incident dementia cases met clinical criteria for AD.[20,34]

This and other population-based reports[42] suggest that AD is by far the most common etiology of dementia. **Figure 2.2** shows the estimated relative proportions of different dementia etiologies observed in the general population and in specialized memory clinics based on the reported literature[43-45] and in my own clinical experience. The prevalence of etiologies in demented patients presenting to private practitioners has not been estimated but would likely reflect intermediate values between these two charts.

FIGURE 2.2 — DIAGNOSIS OF DEMENTIA: POPULATION-BASED VS CLINIC-BASED ESTIMATES

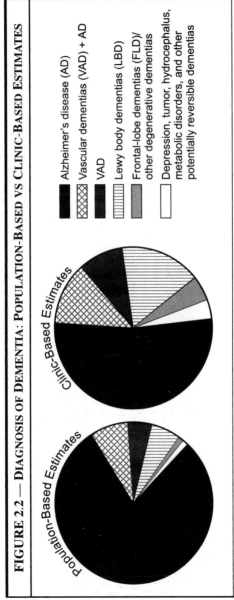

- Alzheimer's disease (AD)
- Vascular dementias (VAD) + AD
- VAD
- Lewy body dementias (LBD)
- Frontal-lobe dementias (FLD)/ other degenerative dementias
- Depression, tumor, hydrocephalus, metabolic disorders, and other potentially reversible dementias

Population-Based Estimates

Clinic-Based Estimates

Data based on: Small GW, et al. *JAMA.* 1997;278:1363-1371; American Psychiatric Association. *Am J Psychiatry.* 1997;154(suppl 5):1-39; Morris JC. *Clin Geriatr Med.* 1994;10:257-276; Drs. Martin Farlow and John Breitner. Personal communication. 1998; and the author's clinical experience.

3

Evaluation of the Older Patient With Cognitive Problems

In a typical health-care setting, there are three ways that patients with possible cognitive impairment may be identified for clinical evaluation and subsequent diagnosis:

- Patient presents to the clinician with a complaint of memory or thinking problems
- Family member or friend brings the patient to the clinician and draws attention to observed cognitive or behavioral problems that the patient confirms, minimizes, or denies
- Clinician or office staff member performs a brief cognitive screening test on a patient without complaints and identifies a possible problem that triggers further evaluation.

Currently, most clinicians do not screen for cognitive problems in their practice unless they receive complaints from either the patient or the patient's family. This is unfortunate since the majority of patients with dementing illnesses do not complain about it to their health-care providers, and on average, family members do not seek medical attention for the patient until several years after the onset of symptoms.

As we enter the age of increasingly effective therapeutic interventions for the most common diseases that produce dementia in older adults (Alzheimer's disease [AD], vascular disease, and depression), a convincing case can be made that:

- It is no longer appropriate to simply offer reassurance without evaluation to patients who complain of memory or other cognitive problems.
- All patients over the age of 65 should be routinely screened for cognitive impairment.
- Once discovered, even mild memory and thinking problems should be evaluated as they may signal a reversible disorder or the early symptoms of a progressive illness affecting cognition that can be treated.
- There are important advantages to early diagnosis of dementing disorders (**Table 3.1**).

Classic symptoms that should raise the suspicion of a dementia syndrome are listed in **Table 3.2**. Yet, symptoms of cognitive impairment should not only be evaluated based upon impairment but also upon whether the patient has experienced a *decline* from his

---

TABLE 3.1 — ADVANTAGES OF EARLY DIAGNOSIS IN DEMENTING CONDITIONS

For Every Case
- Provide a diagnostic answer and education for the patient and/or family.

For Patients With Reversible or Static Diseases
(eg, depression, stroke)
- Relieve the fear of an irreversible or progressive disease.
- Treat the underlying disease.
- Initiate prevention and/or rehabilitation strategies.

For Patients With Irreversible and Progressive Diseases
(eg, Alzheimer's disease)
- Treat cognitive and behavioral symptoms.
- Plan legal and financial future while patient is still competent.
- Initiate management strategies that will postpone dependence and institutionalization.

**TABLE 3.2 — COMMON
SYMPTOMS OF DEMENTIA**

- Memory loss affecting job skills or other activities
- Difficulty performing familiar tasks
- Problems with language
- Disorientation
- Impaired judgment
- Problems with abstract thinking
- Continuous misplacement of personal possessions
- Changes in mood or behavior
- Changes in personality
- Loss of initiative

or her usual level of function. For example, a university professor may complain that he or she can no longer teach a familiar class without notes, while someone working with fewer high-level cognitive demands may not notice problems in the workplace but may neglect paying the bills. Listening to patients and families as they describe declines in cognitive competency will allow much earlier recognition of dementing syndromes.

Regardless of how the patient is identified for evaluation, the process of clinical evaluation emphasizes history, physical and mental status examination, and ancillary diagnostic studies (**Figure 3.1**). The diagnosis of conditions that cause cognitive impairment, including AD, is no longer a process of exclusion but is now one of identifying features consistent with particular diseases. The clinician should also keep in mind that in older patients, it is common to find multiple contributions to cognitive impairment rather than a single cause.

Patient History

Some clinicians attempt to collect historical information solely from the patient, but this is unwise be-

FIGURE 3.1 — ALGORITHM FOR DEMENTIA EVALUATION AND DIAGNOSIS

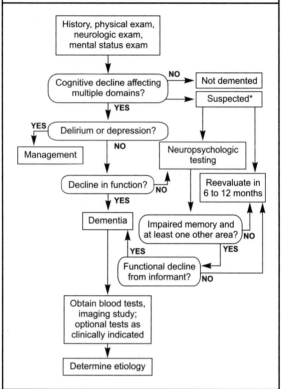

* Worrisome history without obvious mental status deficit or impaired memory only, suggesting mild cognitive impairment (see Chapter 6, *Natural History*).

Modified from: Corey-Bloom J, et al. *Neurology.* 1995;45:211-218.

cause demented persons often minimize or deny their problems, and self-assessments of memory problems do not accurately reflect functional abilities. Therefore, *the history should always be gathered from a family member or close acquaintance, in addition to the patient.* Since family members often defer to inaccurate histories given by patients when both are in the same room, and because patients are reluctant to share their psychological state as freely when a family member is present, *both the patient and a family member or other reliable informant should be interviewed separately.* At the outset, the clinician should investigate the history of:

- Current symptoms and functional capabilities
- Current and prior medical and neuropsychiatric history.

■ Current Symptoms and Functional Capabilities

It is important to distinguish between sudden or insidious onset and slower progression from more acute and subacute disorders. However, the history can sometimes be misleading, as the family's first report of symptoms may be associated with a disorienting vacation, a fever, a minor surgical operation, or other stressful circumstances that may have only unmasked the underlying condition. Family members and other observers may erroneously consider these events to have caused the patient's symptoms, making it difficult to obtain the true history of the onset of the illness.

The course of the symptoms is important as well. Symptoms that include prolonged periods of apparent return to normal, are more likely to represent depression, medication overdoses, or metabolic disorders than symptoms that slowly and progressively decline.

A history that seeks to understand which cognitive domains are impaired can also help with diagnosis. For example, the typical patient with mild AD maintains socially appropriate behavior and conversational style, while the patient with frontal lobe dementia may have problems with social comportment or demonstrate inappropriate social or workplace behavior early in the course of the disease.

A functional history to assess how well patients are successfully maintaining activities of daily living should include information about:

- Work performance (if the patient is still working) or reasons for retirement (if not still working)
- Management of personal finances
- Driving
- Household activities and hobbies
- Dressing, bathing, and preparation of meals.

Asking about recent performance capabilities in these areas not only provides important clues about the degree of impairment but can reveal potential legal, financial, and physical dangers that may require the clinician to intervene. For example, an employed patient with memory problems may be in immediate danger of losing his or her job for poor performance. In this situation, with the patient's permission, proactive intervention by the clinician could prevent termination of employment while the etiology of the problem is being diagnosed and treated. Moreover, a timely diagnosis while the patient is still employed may permit the utilization of disability benefits that would be lost if the condition were diagnosed after employment was terminated. In a more severely impaired patient who is living alone or driving independently, immediate steps may be necessary to intervene in a situation where there is a high risk of financial dissolution, driving accidents, or even insufficient personal care (see Chapter 10, *Family Education and Support*).

■ Current and Prior Medical and Neuropsychiatric History

It is essential to inquire about prior and current medical and neuropsychiatric diseases, particularly those metabolic, neurologic, and psychiatric disorders that could impact cognition. History of head trauma, stroke, sleep apnea, or any neurologic disease is of clear importance. A general medical history and thorough review of systems is also essential to discover concomitant diseases of the liver, kidney, thyroid, or cardiovascular system that, when treated, could result in improvement or even reversal of cognitive impairment. A history of alcohol abuse should be sought. A careful review of medications will frequently reveal dosages or combinations that are unnecessary or inappropriate for the patient's age and that may exacerbate cognitive deficits. Common medications that may have such an effect include most psychoactive medications (hypnotics, anxiolytics, antidepressants), many medications with anticholinergic effects, and some of most of the commonly used medications for blood pressure. (See **Table 4.5** for common medication categories that can impair cognition.)

If a patient is already obviously impaired, a history that includes a more formal functional assessment will be helpful in designing a management strategy for the family. Impairment of functional performance in the dementing diseases is associated with:

- Instrumental activities of daily living (managing finances, telephoning, driving a car, taking medication, planning a meal, shopping, working)
- Activities of daily living (dressing, bathing, toileting, grooming, eating, walking).

The Functional Assessment Questionnaire, an example of one simple scale for evaluating functional abilities, is shown in **Figure 3.2**.

FIGURE 3.2 — FUNCTIONAL ASSESSMENT QUESTIONNAIRE

Informant's name: _____

Patient's name: _____

Date: _____

Instructions: Place a check mark under the column that best describes the patient's ability to perform the tasks listed below.

	Completely unable to perform task (3 points)	Requires assistance (2 points)	Has difficulty but accomplishes task; or has never done, but the informant feels could do task with difficulty (1 point)	Normal performance, or has never done task, but the informant feels the patient could do the task if necessary (0 points)
1. Writing checks, paying bills, balancing a checkbook	—	—	—	—
2. Assembling tax records, business affairs, or papers	—	—	—	—
3. Shopping alone for clothes, household necessities, or groceries	—	—	—	—
4. Playing a game of skill, working on a hobby	—	—	—	—

5. Heating water, making a cup of coffee, turning off the stove	|	|
6. Preparing a balanced meal	|	|
7. Keeping track of current events	|	|
8. Paying attention to, understanding, or discussing a television show, book, or magazine	|	|
9. Remembering appointments, family occasions, holidays, or medications	|	|
10. Traveling out of the neighborhood, driving, arranging to take buses	|	|
Total Points per Column	|	|
		Total Points | |

Adapted from: Pfeffer RI, et al. *J Gerontol.* 1982;37:323-329.

3

Physical Examination

Since so many systemic illnesses can impair cognition or exacerbate an underlying neurologic disease, patients being evaluated for thinking and memory problems should have a comprehensive physical examination and a brief mental status examination. As with any evaluation, the physical examination will be tailored to verifying or disproving hypotheses that have been raised by the history. In particular, the clinician should note:

- Hypertension and signs of vascular disease
- Signs of cardiac disease, particularly features suggestive of increased risk for cerebral emboli
- Signs suggesting pulmonary, endocrine, or connective tissue diseases
- Neurologic abnormalities, such as focal weakness, gait problems, parkinsonism, or myoclonus
- Psychiatric features that suggest depression or thought disorder.

Since many of the etiologies of dementia, including some that are reversible, are associated with distinctive signs on neurologic examination (see Chapter 4, *Dementing Disorders Not Due to Alzheimer's Disease*), there is no substitute for performing at least a brief neurologic examination on every patient with cognitive impairment. Clinicians who are unprepared or unwilling to perform a brief neurologic examination and a brief mental status examination should refer patients with dementing illnesses to other clinicians or specialists.

Mental Status Assessment

Assessing the mental status of patients may be done to achieve one or more of the following goals:

- Screening for cognitive impairment
- Evaluating the patient with self-reported or family-reported cognitive symptoms
- Assessing the severity of an established dementing condition
- Assessing deterioration or improvement over time or as a result of treatment.

These goals can all be accomplished through an informal bedside or office mental status examination[46] or by the administration of one of several simple standardized cognitive rating scales such as the Mini-Mental State Examination (MMSE).

■ Brief Mental Status Evaluation

The bedside or office mental status evaluation should include brief assessments of attention, language, visuospatial function, memory, and executive function. Attention may be measured by asking the patient to perform a nonautomatic sequential task. Examples of attention tests include forward and reverse digit span, serial subtractions (which also measures mental calculation), and reciting the months of the year in reverse. The assessment of attention is particularly important since the remainder of the mental status examination will be nonspecifically impaired by inattention. Also, a clinical presentation marked by pronounced inattention may suggest an entirely different diagnosis than one in which attention is preserved and amnestic deficits are more salient. For example, the subacute development of predominantly attentional symptoms might represent a metabolic encephalopathy.

For the evaluation of language, fluency may be assessed through spontaneous conversation, but there is no substitute for specific examination of comprehension, naming, and repetition.[47] It is particularly important to assess auditory comprehension before making judgments about the patient's ability to follow instructions on the rest of the mental status examination. It is useful to test reading and writing since the relative preservation of these skills that is commonly found in some forms of dementia can be used to help even severely amnestic patients to continue functioning.

Rudimentary visuospatial functions may be assessed by having the patient fill in the numbers of a clock face or copy a complex drawing, although it should be recognized that these tasks also require attention, sequencing, and integration skills. Strokes, as well as some degenerative dementias, may be characterized by early and specific loss of visuospatial abilities, and an awareness of visuospatial deficits may help the clinician to make recommendations about orientation and driving.

Impaired memory is the most common complaint of patients presenting with dementia, even when the primary problem is inattention, since the consolidation of new learning is impaired by attentional deficits. The bedside testing of memory should, at a minimum, include an assessment of the patient's orientation (day, date, season, year, and location), a measure of previously learned material, and a test of new learning (such as spontaneous recall of a list of three to five unrelated words after 5 to 10 minutes of distraction). Previously learned material may be assessed informally by asking for the patient's year of birth, children's names, the names of prior presidents, or recent wars. More recently learned material may be explored by asking about current events. Since confabulation accompanies some memory disorders, care should be taken not to ask for answers that cannot be verified by the clinician or a family member. Short-term memory or new learning is particularly impaired in some forms of dementia, such as AD. The patient of any age with normal memory should be able to learn three items after a single presentation trial and repeat them correctly after 5 to 10 minutes of distraction. However, subtle memory deficits are not always apparent on such simple memory testing and may require more extensive neuropsychologic examination to document.

Each clinician may find it useful to develop his or her own routine battery of mental status testing that may be given to every patient being examined. However, some aspects of the examination, such as reading ability, will be more dependent upon educational level than others, such as attention. Therefore, the clinician must be prepared to temper such methods with sufficient flexibility to test patients of various backgrounds and educational experience. The clinician with special interest in neurobehavioral assessment will wish to extend the mental status testing to include measures of modality-specific memory, praxis, prosody, complex motor movements, and response inhibition.[46]

■ **The Mini-Mental State Examination**

Many clinicians are more comfortable administering a standardized scale to assess cognitive function. An additional advantage of such scales in the busy office environment is that it can be administered by any trained person rather than the clinician himself or herself.

The most commonly used brief cognitive rating scale is the MMSE (**Figure 3.3**),[48] which was originally designed to quickly assess the cognitive state of older psychiatric patients and has since been widely used both to screen for cognitive impairment and to measure the severity of dementia. The MMSE includes 11 questions, requires 5 to 10 minutes and minimal training to administer. The first section calls for verbal responses to assess orientation, memory, and attention. The remaining sections examine simple naming, the ability to follow verbal and written com-

FIGURE 3.3 — MINI-MENTAL STATE EXAMINATION

Patient's Name _____

Date Test Given _____

Score 1 for each blank space. Please tell me the:

____ Year ____ Season ____ Date ____ Day _____ Month ____
____ State ____ County _____ City ____ Location ____ Floor _____

I am going to ask you to remember some words. First listen to me saying them, then say them back to me. (Score the number repeated on the first trial only.) After patient learns all three, tell patient that he/she will be asked to remember these words later.

____ Orange _____ Airplane _____ Tobacco _____
(trials to learn all three items ____)

Subtract 7 from 100 and then subtract 7 from each answer, if patient misses two subtractions, stop. If patient misses one but accurately subtracts 7 from the incorrect answer, score as correct (eg, for 93, 87, 80, 73, 66 score 4).

____ 93 _____ 86 _____ 79 _____ 72 ____ 65 ____

If the patient can't do serial 7s, you can substitute: Spell the word WORLD backwards. Score 1 for each letter given in the correct order even if there is a missing letter (eg, DLRW score 4) or a reversal of two letters (DLORW score 3).

____ D ____ L ____ O ____ R ____ W ____

What were the three words I asked you to remember earlier?

____ Orange _____ Airplane _____ Tobacco _____

Point to and ask the patient to name a:

____ Pencil _____ Watch _____

Repeat the following phrase:

____ No ifs, ands, or buts.

____ Read and obey.   **CLOSE YOUR EYES**

____ Take this piece of paper with your right hand, _____ fold it in half, _____ and drop in on the desk _____ .

____ Copy the following drawing:

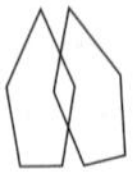

____ Write a sentence.

____ **Total**

Modified from: Folstein MF, et al. *J Psychiatr Res.* 1975;12: 189-198.

mands, to write a sentence spontaneously, and to copy a geometric figure.

There is a maximum possible total score of 30. Originally, scores below 24 were typically interpreted to suggest some degree of dementia,[49] but now it is clear that mild cognitive impairment may be seen with scores as high as 27 in highly educated persons since patients with mild amnestic disorders may have difficulty with spontaneous recall but not with any other items. The MMSE is considered to be well validated,[50] but its sensitivity is considerably diminished for older patients, patients with lower educational levels, and patients with mild but unequivocal dementia.[50-55] Despite these limitations, the MMSE continues to be the single most popular screening test administered by geriatric health-care providers and researchers because of its brevity and ease of administration. **Figure 6.1** in Chapter 6, *Natural History,* illustrates a typical decline in MMSE scores associated with progression of AD.

■ Screening for Depression

Depression is a common problem in older adults, with some estimates of the prevalence as high as 15%,[56] yet depressed older patients may not complain of depression and sometimes vehemently deny depressed mood. Instead, they frequently present with complaints of:

- Somatic symptoms
- Sleep problems
- Memory difficulties.

The clinician can explore these complaints by asking tactful questions about mood and probing for additional vegetative signs, such as loss of interests, appetite, and libido.

Brief standardized scales are also available to screen for depression in patients presenting with memory complaints (**Table 3.3**). For example, the Ge-

TABLE 3.3 — BRIEF SCALES FOR ASSESSING DEPRESSION IN PATIENTS WITH MEMORY COMPLAINTS

Scale	Completed by Clinician	Completed by Patient	Completed by Observer	Quality of Results in Demented Patients
Geriatric Depression Scale (Yesavage 1988[a])	No	Yes	Yes	Adequate
Hamilton Depression Scale (Hamilton 1960[b]; Williams 1988[c])	Yes	No	Yes	Adequate
Cornell Scale for Depression in Dementia (Alexopoulous 1988[d])	Yes	No	No	Preferable
Dementia Mood Assessment Scale (Sunderland 1988[e])	Yes	No	No	Preferable

[a]Yesavage JA. *Psychopharmacol Bull*. 1988;24:709-711; [b]Hamilton M. *J Neurol Neurosurg Psychiatry*. 1960;23:56-61; [c]Williams JB. *Arch Gen Psychiatry*. 1988;45:742-747; [d]Alexopoulos GS, et al. *Biol Psychiatry*. 1988;23:271-284; [e]Sunderland T, et al. *Am J Psychiatry*. 1988;145:955-959.

riatric Depression Scale is a 15- or 30-item self-report questionnaire with a yes/no response format that can be administered in 8 to 10 minutes.[57,58] It should be remembered that there is considerable overlap between the symptoms of depression and those of early degenerative dementias such as AD. For example, in the early stages of most degenerative dementias there is frequently a withdrawal and loss of interest from hobbies and many external activities. Therefore, scores indicating depression on the above scales should always be evaluated in the context of whether they may be indicative of cognitive impairment. Further discussion about diagnosis and treatment of depression presenting as dementia is found in Chapter 4, *Dementing Disorders Not Due to Alzheimer's Disease*.

Ancillary Diagnostic Studies

The history, physical examination, and mental status testing are sufficient to make a confident diagnosis in most patients with a classic presentation of AD. However, some ancillary studies are routinely recommended and others are occasionally recommended when there is diagnostic uncertainty. The more experienced the practitioner and the more clear-cut the diagnostic possibilities, the more specific the choices of ancillary tests can be. Choices of ancillary studies may also be affected by reimbursement protocols and the development of new screening tests. For example, biologic markers in blood, urine, and cerebrospinal fluid have been marketed with largely unsupported claims that they can assist in the diagnosis of AD. These are discussed in greater detail in Chapter 5, *Risk Factors, Genetics, Biomarkers, and Diagnostic Accuracy*.

In cases where the diagnosis is clear from the history and physical examination, the goal of ancillary studies is to screen for occult superimposed medical or neurologic disorders. For example, in a patient with classic AD, it would still be important to discover an unsuspected depression, metabolic abnormality, infection, or stroke.

Recommendations for laboratory and imaging studies in patients when the primary etiology of the dementia is clear include:

- Complete blood count and blood chemistries (including sodium, potassium, calcium, phosphate, liver function tests, creatinine, thyroid stimulating hormone), B_{12} level, Venereal Disease Research Laboratory [test for syphilis] (VDRL), and sedimentation rate
- At least one computed tomography (CT) or magnetic resonance imaging (MRI) scan without contrast. Since the sensitivity of the MRI is so much greater than the CT, MRI is preferred whenever possible.

The evaluation of atypical dementias defies formulaic recommendations since there are so many neurologic and psychiatric diseases that can affect cognition (**Table 4.1** and **Table 4.2**). In general, when the primary etiology of the dementia is not clear, referral to a neurologist, neuropsychiatrist, or geriatric psychiatrist should be considered, along with the following studies:

- Referral to a neuropsychologist for formal cognitive testing
- MRI scan with contrast
- Additional laboratory tests
- Lumbar puncture
- Electroencephalography or polysomnography
- Functional imaging
- Brain biopsy.

■ Neuropsychologic Evaluation

Patient evaluation and psychometric testing by a neuropsychologist have become the accepted clinical standard for the detailed characterization of cognitive deficits. While neuropsychologic testing is not necessary for the proper evaluation of every patient with dementia, it is invaluable in the very early stages of the condition and in the complex or the atypical patient. It is also useful for following subtle deterioration or improvement in a given patient over time or after treatment.

It should be pointed out that the bedside mental status examination previously described is drawn almost entirely from the more extensive forms of testing that have been developed within the relatively new field of neuropsychology. A detailed discussion of neuropsychologic testing in aging and dementia is beyond the scope of this manual but is readily available from other sources.[59-62]

Appropriate referral to a neuropsychologist for testing and evaluation is extremely valuable in order to:

- Assist with the diagnosis of very mild or atypical presentations
- Obtain scores that can help decide issues of competency and independence around contested issues of self-care, finances, and driving
- Establish a careful baseline of cognitive abilities from which to measure declines or improvements over time.

■ Structural Imaging Studies

Simple atrophy on structural images is not usually helpful in the evaluation of individual patients with dementia because of the overlap between brain atrophy that occurs in normal aging with the more pronounced atrophy that is usually present in the degenerative dementias. Focal atrophy in the para-hippocampal region may have diagnostic value for early AD,[63-66] but the use of this is currently limited to specialized centers that apply standardized procedures for scanning and measurement.

Magnetic resonance imaging scans of older patients frequently reveal scattered or extensive bright signals in the cerebral white matter on T2 scans, without corresponding loss of tissue on T1 scans. The neuropathology corresponding to these white-matter hyperintensities (WMH—also called leukoaraiosis) is variable; they have been associated with small infarctions, gliosis and demyelination, cerebral amyloid angiopathy, and periventricular venous collagenosis.[67-69] In the routine clinical evaluation of dementia, a small amount of WMH probably has little diagnostic significance. However, extensive WMH appears to be a risk factor for stroke, gait deterioration, and depression. Therefore, extensive WMH may represent cerebrovascular lesions or other neurologic diseases affecting white matter (**Figure 4.1**).

Structural imaging (preferably MRI scan) is most useful in the workup of dementia in order to discover:
- Small or large strokes
- Hydrocephalus
- Tumors
- Focal or generalized atrophy
- Clues to rare conditions, such as white matter diseases, vasculitis, carcinomatous meningitis, or cerebral infections.

■ **Additional Laboratory Blood Tests**

Depending upon the history and examination, some additional tests to consider include calcium, phosphorus, zinc, magnesium, copper and ceruloplasmin, amylase, cholestanol, cortisol, serum pH, arterial blood gases, human immunodeficiency virus, antiphospholipid antibodies, antineuronal antibodies, and urinalysis.

■ Lumbar Puncture and Analysis of Cerebrospinal Fluid

Lumbar puncture and examination of the cerebrospinal fluid (CSF) are not necessary in the vast majority of patients who are evaluated for dementia. However, in patients younger than 60 years old—and in anyone who has history, signs, symptoms, or laboratory studies suggestive of hydrocephalus, infection, vasculitis, or cancer—lumbar puncture should be considered. Spinal fluid tests to be considered would include evaluation of CSF pressure, cell count, and differential, bacterial, and fungal cultures, VDRL, cryptococcal antibody, tau, and amyloid beta peptide$_{42}$. The current and future role of CSF evaluation in the development of screening and diagnostic tests for specific dementias such as AD is considered further in Chapter 5, *Risk Factors, Genetics, Biomarkers, and Diagnostic Accuracy*.

■ Electroencephalography and Polysomnography

An electroencephalogram (EEG) is not useful for the routine diagnostic evaluation of cognitive impairment in older persons. The most salient reasons to obtain an EEG would be in cases where Creutzfeldt-Jakob disease (CJD) is suspected (see discussion of CJD in Chapter 4, *Dementing Disorders Not Due to Alzheimer's Disease*)[70,71] and in some unusual situations where it is necessary to rule out seizures, encephalitis, and metabolic abnormalities.

Occasionally, older patients with sleep apnea can present with confusional states and cognitive impairment, usually in conjunction with extreme daytime sleepiness. Polysomnography with monitoring of oxygenation and respiration can uncover the diagnosis of treatable sleep apnea.

■ Functional Imaging Studies

Cerebral blood flow reflects the metabolic status of the brain and can be considerably more sensitive to early dementing diseases than structural images.[72] Regional blood flow can be visualized using single photon emission CT,[73] while positron emission tomography (PET) can provide more direct regional measures of glucose or oxygen metabolism. Although not routinely performed in the evaluation of dementia, these modalities can yield important diagnostic information in early or atypical cases by providing regional profiles of blood flow or metabolic activity in the brain, particularly when used in conjunction with information derived from neuropsychologic testing and structural imaging (**Figure 4.2** and **Color Plate 1**).[74,75] For example, a pattern of bilateral temporoparietal hypoperfusion or hypometabolism is characteristic of AD, and while this pattern may not be seen in all individuals with early cases of AD,[76-78] groups at greater and lesser risk for AD can be differentiated by both fMRI and PET studies (**Color Plate 1**).[79,80] A recent research finding of considerable interest is the development of an amyloid-imaging PET tracer that appears to be retained and imaged in areas of living human brain where large amounts of amyloid would be expected in AD patients (**Color Plate 2**).[81] Similar efforts are underway to image tangle burden.[82] A full review of PET studies and dementia is beyond the scope of this manual, but may be found elsewhere.[75,83,84]

In the future, when combined with other information such as apolipoprotein E genotyping, PET may be capable of detecting early cerebral dysfunction in at-risk persons, even prior to neuropsychologic abnormalities,[72,80,85] and may eventually prove helpful in predicting the rate of cognitive decline in AD.[86] Functional imaging may be used to point to the recruitment of additional neurologic networks in persons with mild disease,[87] to guide brain biopsy,[88] or to provide important information in uncommon cases such as frontal lobe dementia[89] or dementia with combined cognitive and extrapyramidal symptomatology;[90] however, until recently, it has not been recommended for routine use in the diagnostic evaluation of a dementing patient. Fluorodeoxyglucose-positron emission tomography (FDG-PET) is now covered by Medicare *only* in patients who have a documented clinical decline of at least 6 months and a recently established diagnosis of dementia, and who meet diagnostic criteria for both AD *and* frontotemporal dementia (FTD), and in whom the clinical diagnosis is still unclear after conventional evaluation (see http://www.cms.hhs.gov/mcd/viewdecisionmemo.asp?id=104).

■ Brain Biopsy

Brain biopsy is occasionally utilized in the evaluation of an extremely atypical dementia, particularly when a vasculitis or infectious etiology is suspected.[91,92] Discovering a previously unsuspected diagnosis with brain biopsy in a dementia patient is unusual, and even in specialized centers, this procedure is rarely used.

44

4

Dementing Disorders Not Due to Alzheimer's Disease

Despite conflicting data on the prevalence of different etiologies of dementia, particularly from other countries, there is broad consensus that the most common etiology of dementia in the United States is Alzheimer's disease (AD). As described in Chapter 2, *Epidemiology of Dementia*, and illustrated in **Figure 2.2**, AD is so commonly the diagnosis that when confronted with cognitive impairment in older persons, it would be easy for clinicians to routinely make this diagnosis without systematically considering alternative or additional diagnoses, particularly since there is better recognition that truly reversible dementias are relatively infrequent.[93] While such a practice would save time and be correct much of the time by chance, it would do patients with other or additional conditions a great disservice by failing to detect reversible diseases affecting cognition and failing to provide accurate prognoses and family risk information.

As listed in **Table 4.1** and **Table 4.2**, there are dozens of unusual causes of dementing diseases in older individuals that should be considered based on the clues provided in the history and examination. However, the following conditions are relatively common, either alone or in combination with other etiologies, and a brief discussion of each is presented in this chapter:

- Depression
- Overmedication
- Metabolic and endocrine abnormalities
- Vascular dementia (VaD) and mixed dementias

TABLE 4.1 — POTENTIALLY REVERSIBLE CAUSES OF DEMENTIAS

Neoplasms
- Gliomas
- Meningiomas
- Metastatic tumors, carcinoma, lymphoma, leukemia
- Remote effects of carcinomas

Metabolic Disorders
- Thyroid disease (hyper- and hypothyroidism)
- Hypoglycemia
- Hypernatremia and hyponatremia
- Hypercalcemia
- Renal failure
- Hepatic failure
- Cushing's disease
- Addison's disease
- Hypopituitarism
- Wilson's disease

Trauma
- Craniocerebral trauma
- Acute and chronic subdural hematoma

Toxins
- Alcoholism
- Heavy metals (lead, manganese, mercury, arsenic)
- Organic poisons, including solvents and insecticides

Infection
- Bacterial meningitis and encephalitis
- Parasitic meningitis and encephalitis
- Fungal meningitis and encephalitis
- Cryptococcal meningitis
- Viral meningitis and encephalitis
- Brain abscess
- Neurosyphilis: meningovascular, tabes dorsalis, general paresis
- Primary AIDS encephalopathy

Autoimmune Disorders
- Central nervous system vasculitis, temporal arteritis
- Disseminated lupus erythematosus
- Multiple sclerosis

Drugs
- Antidepressants
- Antianxiety agents
- Hypnotics
- Sedatives
- Antiarrhythmics
- Antihypertensives
- Anticonvulsants
- Cardiac medications, including digitalis
- Drugs with anticholinergic effects

Nutritional Disorders
- Thiamine deficiency (Wernicke's encephalopathy and Wernicke-Korsakoff syndrome)
- Vitamin B_{12} deficiency (pernicious anemia)
- Folate deficiency
- Vitamin B_6 deficiency (pellagra)

Psychiatric Disorders
- Depression
- Schizophrenia
- Mania
- Other psychoses

Other Disorders
- Normal-pressure hydrocephalus
- Whipple's disease
- Sarcoidosis
- Sleep apnea

Modified from: Terry RD. *Aging and the Brain*. New York, NY: Lippincott-Raven Publishers; 1988:17-82.

TABLE 4.2 — IRREVERSIBLE CAUSES OF DEMENTIAS

Degenerative Diseases
- Alzheimer's disease
- Frontotemporal dementias
- Huntington's disease
- Progressive supranuclear palsy
- Parkinson's disease
- Diffuse Lewy body disease
- Olivopontocerebellar atrophy
- Amyotrophic lateral sclerosis/parkinsonism-dementia complex
- Hallervorden-Spatz disease
- Kufs' disease
- Wilson's disease (if not treated early enough)
- Metachromatic leukodystrophy
- Adrenoleukodystrophy

Vascular Dementias
- Multiple small or large infarcts
- Binswanger's disease
- Cerebral embolism
- Arteritis
- Anoxia secondary to cardiac arrest, cardiac failure, or carbon monoxide intoxication

Traumatic Dementia
- Craniocerebral injury
- Dementia pugilistica

Infections
- Creutzfeldt-Jakob disease (subacute spongiform encephalopathy)
- Progressive multifocal leukoencephalopathy
- Postencephalitic dementia

Modified from: Terry RD. *Aging and the Brain*. New York, NY: Lippincott-Raven Publishers; 1988:17-82.

- Parkinson's disease (PD) and parkinsonian syndromes
- Lewy body diseases (LBDs)
- Frontotemporal dementias
- Prion diseases and the spongiform encephalopathies
- Huntington's disease
- Dementia associated with human immunodeficiency virus (HIV) infection.

Depression

Depression is common among the elderly. Disturbances of thinking and memory frequently accompany depression[94,95] and have led to the use of the misleading term "pseudodementia." Since depression causes authentic, albeit reversible, cognitive deficits, a more appropriate designation that emphasizes the syndromic nature of the term "dementia" would be the dementia of depression or perhaps depression-related cognitive dysfunction.[96,97]

Confirming the diagnosis of depression in a patient presenting with cognitive impairment can be difficult since the patient may not complain of classic mood changes or vegetative features. Some clinical features can be helpful, although none are diagnostic, and frequent exceptions and overlaps exist (**Table 4.3**). It should be remembered that degenerative brain diseases, such as AD, often coexist with depression in the same patient and that antidepressant treatment can frequently improve mood and quality of life in these patients.

Since depression in the elderly may present atypically and may worsen the cognitive impairments that are already present due to underlying neurodegenerative disease, it is not always easily recognizable and many clinicians maintain an appropriate readiness to

Feature	Depression Presenting as Memory Difficulties	Classic Alzheimer's Disease Without Depression
Age of onset	Common below and above age 60	Rare below age 60
Onset	Subacute or insidious	Insidious
Course of symptoms	Some fluctuations	Progressive decline
Memory complaints	Almost always aware	Sometimes aware, often untroubled by memory
Affective state	Sad or stoic	Sad, stoic, or cheerful
Sleep-wake cycle	Often disturbed	Sometimes disturbed
Language/praxis symptoms and signs	Uncommon unless depression is severe	Uncommon in mild stages, but common in moderate and severe stages
Memory testing	Performs better than self-expectation	Performs worse than self-expectation
Response to cholinesterase inhibitor therapy	Improvement in cognitive status not expected	Modest improvement in cognitive status can occur
Response to antidepressant therapy	Significant improvement likely	Mild improvement in mood or behavior may occur

TABLE 4.3 — SIMILARITIES AND DIFFERENCES IN THE CLINICAL PRESENTATIONS OF DEPRESSION AND EARLY ALZHEIMER'S DISEASE

try antidepressants empirically or even as a therapeutic challenge to evaluate the response. A 6- to 8-week treatment trial of one of the serotonin reuptake inhibitors is relatively safe and sometimes provides considerable and even unexpected improvement. In our clinical experience, an impressive improvement in mood or anxiety may be seen with antidepressant treatment, while the cognitive impairment remains relatively unchanged.

An overview of current antidepressant therapies for the elderly is provided in **Table 4.4**. As a general rule, clinicians should avoid using the medications with significant anticholinergic properties, since older and demented individuals are more sensitive to anticholinergic side effects, such as confusion.

Overmedication

As with depression, cognitive impairments due to sedating or psychoactive medications are often superimposed upon other dementing disorders. Removing or reducing unnecessary medications may improve cognition, even in patients with other diseases, such as AD. Clinicians should be particularly vigilant when evaluating patients who are on sleeping medications, antianxiety medications, and anticholinergic medications.

While many medications can have idiosyncratic effects, **Table 4.5** is a partial list of medication categories that commonly impair cognition. At conventional doses, many medications in these categories may not impair cognition in young patients or even in healthy older individuals but may worsen the cognitive status of older patients who are demented from other causes and who have reduced neurologic reserve.

TABLE 4.4 — CHARACTERISTICS OF SELECTED ANTIDEPRESSANT DRUGS USED IN THE ELDERLY

Generic/(Trade) Drug Name	Initial Daily Dose	Target Dose*	Maximal Dose*	Sedative Effect	Antichol Effect	Postural Hypotens	GI Upset	Sexual Dysfunc
Bupropion (Wellbutrin)	75-100 mg qd	75-100 mg tid	450 mg	0	0	0	++	0
Citalopram (Celexa)	10 mg qd	20-40 mg qd	60 mg	0	0	0	++	++
Desipramine (Norpramin)	10-25 mg qd	75-150 mg qd	300 mg	+	+	++	+	+
Doxepin (Sinequan)	10-25 mg qhd	75-150 mg qhs	300 mg	++++	+++	+++	+	+
Duloxetine (Cymbalta)	20 mg qd-bid	20-30 mg qd-bid	60 mg	++	++	0	++	++
Escitalopram (Lexapro)	10 mg qd	10-20 mg qd	20 mg	0	0	0	++	++
Fluoxetine (Prozac)	10 mg qod-qd	10-30 mg qd	60 mg	0	0	0	++	++
Mirtazapine (Remeron)	15 mg qd	30-45 mg qd	45 mg	+++	+	0	0	+
Nortriptyline (Pamelor)	10-20 mg qhs	25-75 mg qhs	200 mg	++	++	+	+	+
Paroxetine (Paxil)	10-20 mg qd	20-40 mg qd	100 mg	+	0	0	++	++

Sertraline (Zoloft)	25 mg qd	50-100 mg qd	200 mg	0	0	0	++	++
Trazodone (Desyrel)	25 mg qhs	75-200 mg qhs	400 mg	+++	0	++	+	+
Venlafaxine (Effexor)	37.5 mg qd-bid	75-100 mg tid	375 mg	+	+	0	+	++

Abbreviations: antichol, anticholinergic; bid, twice daily; dysfunc, dysfunction; GI, gastrointestinal; hypotens, hypotension; qd, every day; qhs, every night; qod, every other day; tid, three times daily.

* These are dosage recommendations for young and middle-aged adults. Older adults and patients with coexisting neurologic diseases often require lower doses.

0 = no effect to ++++ = frequent effect.

Modified from: Fihn SD, DeWitt DE. *Outpatient Medicine.* 2nd ed. Philadelphia, Pa: WB Saunders Company; 1998.

Metabolic and Endocrine Abnormalities

While metabolic and endocrine abnormalities are not common as isolated causes of cognitive impairment in older adults, they may cause confusional states and, like overmedication, worsen the cognitive status of patients with other etiologies. Common disorders in this category include:

- Hypothyroidism
- Low levels of B_{12}
- Low or high levels of sodium, potassium, calcium, phosphorus
- Hepatic failure
- Renal failure
- Low PO_2
- Serum acidosis or alkalosis.

Treatment of these disorders is generally straightforward and specific to the abnormality and the underlying disease causing it.

There are a number of rare inherited metabolic disorders that are of importance since they can in some instances be treated or even reversed. These include Wilson's disease, Hallervorden-Spatz disease, Fahr's syndrome, peroxisomal disorders, lipoprotein disorders, lipidosis, mitochondrial disorders, adult lysosomal diseases (particularly metachromatic leukodystrophy), adult polyglucosand body disease, Lafora's disease, and neuronal intranuclear hyaline inclusion disease. The presence of these diseases will almost always be signaled by dementia at a younger age and by the accompaniment of neurologic signs such as pyramidal tract signs, extrapyramidal signs, cerebellar signs, ophthalmoplegia, cataracts, visual failure, epilepsy, or peripheral neuropathy.

Vascular Dementia and Mixed Dementias

Vascular dementia (VaD) is considered by many to be the second most common etiology of cognitive decline in the elderly. In the United States, the proportion of demented patients with VaD and mixed dementia with VaD has been most commonly estimated to be between 5% and 35%,[20,98] while some studies from Scandinavian and Asian countries have suggested that VaD may be much more common there, on the order of 30% to 60%.[16,23] Estimates of the prevalence and incidence of VaD are generally lower in population-based studies than in hospital- and practice-based studies.

A diagnosis of VaD requires three essential elements:

- Cognitive impairment or dementia
- Presence of cerebrovascular disease
- Establishment of a causal link between the dementia and the cerebrovascular disease.

In practice, the third element can be problematic because both cognitive impairment and cerebrovascular disease are common, and it can be difficult to confidently establish the causal link between the two. The diagnosis of VaD is further complicated by the wide variety of clinical syndromes that can arise from large or small strokes in various regions of grey or white matter in the brain and by the common co-occurrence of cerebrovascular disease and other forms of dementia, particularly AD. VaD may perhaps best be characterized as a pathophysiologic spectrum with intellectual impairment due to single or multiple brain infarcts at one end and insidiously progressive diffuse small-vessel pathology at the other.[99,100]

On one end of this spectrum are clinically apparent infarcts causing dementia, often described by the diagnostic term "multi-infarct dementia" (MID). When confusion, aphasia, neglect, or memory problems begin suddenly or with a clinically evident stroke, this diagnosis is usually clear. Risk factors for MID are similar to those for clinical stroke and include older age, nonwhite race, history of myocardial infarction, recent cigarette smoking, diabetes, hypertension, and lower educational attainment.[101,102] The likelihood of MID in a specific patient has been estimated with a specific set of questions about the patient's history and examination, designated as an "ischemic score."[103-106] The ischemic score is still useful, although it antedated magnetic resonance imaging (MRI) scans, which are far more sensitive to ischemic brain injury than a clinical history of stroke.

At the other end of the spectrum from clinically apparent infarcts are silent infarcts, especially small lacunar infarcts and subcortical ischemic vascular disease.[100,107] Since the temporal course of these phenomena is not clinically apparent and since they may be discovered only through MRI scanning or even at autopsy, the link to cognitive impairment is frequently unclear. When infarcts or extensive subcortical ischemic vascular disease are imaged on brain scans in patients who also meet clinical criteria for AD, the possibility of a mixed dementia (AD plus VaD) is raised. However, it is often unclear whether the vascular disease is directly causal, contributory, or only coincidental, and in the absence of a definitive biomarker for AD, there are no clinical methods currently available to determine this. When attempts have been made to separate VaD and mixed VaD-AD dementias using neuropathology from autopsy series, pure VaD has been estimated to account for 15% to 19% of dementias and mixed VaD-AD to account for 9% to 18%.[108]

Attempts to develop clinical criteria for VaD have included the NINDS-AIREN criteria (**Table 4.6**)[109] as well as others.[110,111] Criteria for VaD are only moderately accurate because of the difficulty in distinguishing VaD from other coexisting degenerative dementias.[112] Nevertheless, there is evidence to suggest that the presence of small-vessel cerebrovascular disease may worsen the clinical expression of any given pathologic burden of AD.[113]

A particularly confusing area is the dementia associated with small-vessel disease, presumably hypertensive arteriopathy that produces extensive white-matter ischemia (previously called subcortical arteriosclerotic encephalopathy or Binswanger's disease, and now generally referred to as subcortical ischemic VaD). **Figure 4.1** illustrates varying degrees of white-matter change or leukoaraiosis on MRI scan, ranging from mild to extensive; however, the pathologic significance of even severe white-matter leukoaraiosis in cases of dementia is not clear. White matter abnormalities on MRI scans clearly increase with age, but remain of unclear clinical significance. Some are associated pathologically with benign

TABLE 4.6 — DIAGNOSTIC CRITERIA FOR ISCHEMIC VASCULAR DEMENTIA

Essential Requirements
- Dementia involving memory failure and other cognitive functions that interfere with function in daily living
- Cerebrovascular disease (determined through history, examination, or brain imaging)
- Evidence that the above are causally related; features that support causality include:
  - Temporal relationship between stroke and dementia
  - Abrupt or stepwise deterioration in mental function or fluctuating course
  - Specific brain imaging findings, indicating damage to regions important for higher cerebral function

Supportive Clinical Features
- History of cerebrovascular risk factors (eg, hypertension, diabetes mellitus, cardiac disease, elevated cholesterol, smoking)
- Early appearance of gait disturbance or history of frequent falls
- Early appearance of urinary incontinence, not explained by urologic disease
- Frontal lobe or extrapyramidal features (especially common in Binswanger's disease)
- Pseudobulbar features with or without emotional incontinence (occasional "pathologic crying")

Adapted from: Roman GC, et al. *Neurology*. 1993;43:250-260.

FIGURE 4.1 — MAGNETIC RESONANCE IMAGING SCANS OF LEUKOARAIOSIS

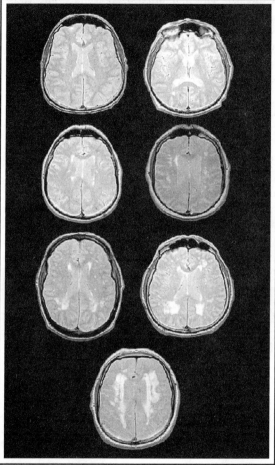

These magnetic resonance imaging scans from seven different patients show increasing amounts of leukoaraiosis in each subsequent image. These white-matter hyperintensities do not represent frank infarcts but may be associated with underlying cerebrovascular pathology.

Photograph courtesy of Dr Charles DeCarli.

perivascular spaces and probably do not influence neurological or cognitive function.[114] However, others are associated with myelin rarefaction, focal gliosis and neuropil atrophy.[115,116] In most studies, white matter abnormalities are associated with cognitive impairment and specific neuropsychological features (impaired attention, executive function, and motor performance) have been associated with these lesions.[107,117-119]

Amyloid angiopathy is a specific form of vascular amyloidosis that affects only the cerebral vasculature without systemic vascular amyloid deposits.[120,121] Cerebral amyloid angiopathy (CAA) can be found in 30% to 50% of random samples of older brains and in association with 80% to 90% of cases that have AD neuropathology. CAA is a common cause of spontaneous lobar hemorrhage in elderly patients and can also cause a rapidly progressive dementing syndrome without hemorrhage, in the absence of typical neuropathology of AD.[122] The dementia associated with CAA generally progresses over days or weeks and is often accompanied by focal or transient neurologic features, including seizures. In addition to severe vascular amyloid, the pathology of CAA dementia can include large and small cortical hemorrhages, small cortical infarctions, white-matter destruction, and neuritic plaques. The pathological presence of CAA is associated with the ε4 allele of the APOE polymorphism, but the ε2 allele is most strongly associated with CAA hemorrhage and recurrence of CAA-related hemorrhages.[123-125]

The syndrome of cerebral autosomal dominant arteriopathy with subcortical infarcts and leucoencephalopathy (CADASIL) is a monogenic cause of stroke, small-vessel disease, and dementia in middle aged persons.[126,127] The clinical features of CADASIL include strokes and transient ischemic attacks, cognitive impairment, migraines with aura, psychiatric disorders and seizures, and the MR scan shows diffuse white matter abnormalities and lacunar infarcts. The disease is caused by mutations in the NOTCH3 gene coding for a large transmembrane receptor in vascular smooth muscle cells, and the underlying pathology is a unique non-amyloid angiopathy that can be determined by skin biopsy.[128,129]

Treatments for typical VaD focus on the reduction of stroke risk factors, such as hypertension, and prevention of further vascular damage with antithrombotic therapies (antiplatelet and anticoagulation medications). There is also preliminary evidence that treating hypertension decreases the likelihood of developing dementia of all types, including AD.[130] At the present time, there is some evidence to suggest that patients with VaD will benefit from anticholinesterase therapies,[131-133] and from memantine,[134-136] although these medications are not approved for that condition.

Parkinson's Disease and Parkinsonian Syndromes

Studies of early-onset PD patients suggest that even nondemented PD patients have mild cognitive changes.[137,138] When PD patients are followed over at least 8 years, more than three-quarters of them develop dementia,[139] and even when motor symptoms respond to dopamine supplementation, the cognitive symptoms do not. Patients with PD who have cognitive deficits are likely to be older and to have:

- Familial or late-onset PD
- More severe symptoms of bradykinesia and postural instability (rather than tremor)
- Depression
- Psychosis or confusion with levodopa treatment
- Earlier mortality from PD.

Depression, which is particularly common in PD (associated perhaps with the loss of norepinephrine neurons in the locus ceruleus), may complicate the assessment of cognitive deficits in such patients. Similarly, anticholinergic medication often used in the treatment of PD may exacerbate a patient's cognitive difficulties.

Lewy bodies (see below) define the classic pathology of PD. But Lewy bodies are also commonly found in AD brains, and the brains of patients with PD sometimes show Alzheimer-like pathology. The spectrum of LBDs is discussed in the next section. The features of dementia in PD are very similar to the features of dementia in LBD.[140]

In addition to PD and LBD, a number of other parkinsonian or Parkinson-plus syndromes are accompanied by dementia (**Table 4.7**). These syndromes are generally not responsive to dopamine supplementation.

Lewy Body Diseases

Lewy bodies are eosinophilic cytoplasmic inclusions with pale haloes that are found within neurons. In patients with PD, Lewy bodies are found in specific brain-stem nuclei. In some diseases, they may be distributed more widely throughout the brain, including the cortex. There is considerable controversy about the definition of dementia associated with LBDs, but one current nosology, emphasizing pathologic findings, divides these diseases into:

- Idiopathic PD
- Diffuse Lewy body disease (DLBD), without prominent neuritic plaques or neurofibrillary tangles
- Lewy body variant of AD.

TABLE 4.7 — DEMENTIA SYNDROMES WITH DISTINCTIVE NEUROLOGIC FEATURES							
Neurologic Feature	Parkinson's Disease	Progressive Supranuclear Palsy	Olivoponto-cerebellar Degeneration	Corticobasal Ganglionic Degeneration	Striatonigral Degeneration	Shy-Drager Syndrome	Lewy Body Diseases
Bradykinesia, rigidity, and postural instability	+++	+++	++	++	+++	++	++
Dementia	++	++	+	++	+	+	+++
Tremor	+++	+	+	+	+	+	+
Apraxia	+	+	+	+++	+	+	+
Gaze palsy	+	+++	0	0	+	0	0
Pyramidal signs	0	+	0	0	++	0	0
Cerebellar signs	0	+	+++	+	+	+	0
Motor response to levodopa	+++	+	0	+	+	+	+
Hallucinations	+	+	+	+	+	+	++
Autonomic impairment	+	0	+	0	++	+++	+
0 = features are absent; + = minimally present; ++ = moderately present; +++ = prominently present.							

63

Some investigators consider LBDs to be a spectrum that includes PD at one end and DLBD at the other.[141,142] Between the two ends lie the great majority of DLBD brains, many of which also have AD pathology. Broad variation in the clinical spectrum also exists, so that each patient can have a slightly different combination of parkinsonism, dementia, tremor, and dystonia. However, taken together, DLBD represents a common pathologic correlate of cognitive impairment in the elderly, perhaps exceeding the prevalence of VaD. Specific pathologic and clinical features have been proposed for LBD (**Table 4.8**).[143-145]

Lewy body disease patients will typically have mental status impairment with increased tone and parkinsonian features, along with a fluctuating clinical course, hallucinations, and behavioral problems, but clinical diagnostic accuracy is low.[143,146-148] When both parkinsonian symptoms and cognitive impairment exist in the same patient, there is often an overlap of diagnostic terminology. If the movement-disorders symptoms predominate, such patients are often characterized as PD with dementia and treated with anticholinergic medications or levodopa, which can cause their cognitive status to worsen and exacerbate their hallucinations. If cognitive symptoms predominate, particularly with hallucinations or delusions, such patients may be treated with neuroleptics, which can cause their extrapyramidal symptoms to worsen.

Designing medication treatment protocols for patients with LBD is challenging because of the simultaneous presence of motor, behavioral, and cognitive problems. As noted above, medications that improve symptoms in one of these areas may worsen them in other areas. However, there is some preliminary evidence that dementia associated with LBDs may be responsive to cholinesterase inhibitors (Chapter 8, *Current and Emerging Therapies*), and an empiric trial

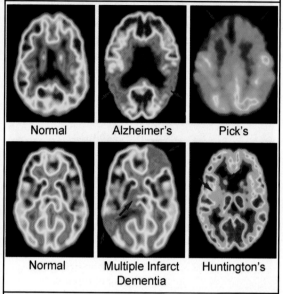

COLOR PLATE 1 — GLUCOSE METABOLIC PATTERNS IN DEMENTIA

Normal

Alzheimer's

Pick's

Normal

Multiple Infarct Dementia

Huntington's

Fluorodeoxyglucose–positron emission tomography (FDG-PET) images show distinctive patterns of hypometabolism in different dementing diseases.

Photos courtesy of Gary Small, MD, UCLA School of Medicine.

COLOR PLATE 2 — AMYLOID-IMAGING PET

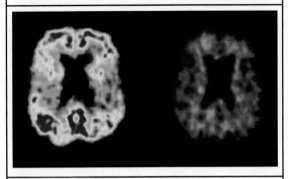

(Left) Amyloid-imaging positron emission tomography (PET) tracer is retained in the cortex of a patient with Alzheimer's disease in areas known to contain large amounts of amyloid. *(Right)* Amyloid-imaging PET is not retained in the cortex of an age-matched control subject.

This experimental technology uses the Pittsburgh Compound-B (PIB) to illuminate amyloid in the brain and may be useful soon in early diagnosis or in tracking the impact of treatments on amyloid in the brain.

Photos courtesy of Bill Klunk, MD, University of Pittsburgh School of Medicine.[181]

TABLE 4.8 — CONSENSUS GUIDELINES FOR THE DIAGNOSIS OF LEWY BODY DISEASE

The central feature required for the diagnosis of Lewy body disease (LBD) is progressive cognitive decline of sufficient magnitude to interfere with normal or occupational function. Prominent or persistent memory impairment may not necessarily occur in the early stages but is usually evident with progression.

- Core features:
  - Fluctuating cognition with pronounced variations in attention and alertness
  - Recurrent visual hallucinations that are typically well formed and detailed
  - Spontaneous motor features of parkinsonism:
    - Two of the core features are essential for the diagnosis of probable LBD
    - One of the core features is essential for the diagnosis of possible LBD
- Features supportive of the diagnosis:
  - Repeated falls
  - Syncope
  - Transient loss of consciousness
  - Neuroleptic sensitivity
  - Systematized delusions
  - Hallucinations in other modalities
- A diagnosis of LBD is less likely in the presence of:
  - Stroke disease, evident as focal neurologic signs or on brain imaging
  - Evidence on physical examination and investigation of any physical illness or other brain disorder sufficient to account for the clinical picture

McKeith IG, et al. *Neurology*. 1996;47:1113-1124.

of these is usually warranted.[149,150] The behavioral symptoms in LBD are best treated with newer "atypical" antipsychotic medications that have minimal extrapyramidal side effects (Chapter 9, *Management of Agitation and Behavioral Symptoms*).

Frontotemporal Dementias

The frontotemporal dementias (FTDs) are a pathologically heterogeneous group of disorders characterized by distinctive behavioral, cognitive, and neuroimaging patterns.[151-153] Diagnostic criteria have been published[154-156] but the clinical features can vary depending upon the relative involvement of the frontal and temporal lobes, and many patients with FTD also meet NINCDS-ADRDA criteria for AD.[157] These disorders may be present in 10% to 25% of dementia cases, and in nearly 50% of cases presenting in persons <65 years of age.[158,159] FTDs can begin as early as the fifth decade and may be distinguished from AD by some or all of the following[160]:

- Social and interpersonal disinhibition with inappropriate and antisocial behaviors
- Apathy, abulia, and reduced initiative
- Compulsions, including hyperorality
- Relative preservation of memory and visuospatial skills
- Aphasia, echolalia, and other language deficits, progressing to mutism.

Approximately 40% of all FTD cases show a familial pattern,[161] usually autosomal dominant inheritance, and a number of distinct mutations in the tau gene, linked to chromosome 17, have been reported,[162,163] but tau mutations appear not to account for all of the familial forms of FTD.[164] Genetic testing and counseling for FTD can be offered.[165]

The terminology used to describe the FTDs is changing. Pick bodies are argentophilic cytoplasmic structures, made up of tau isoforms with different phosphorylation patterns than the tau found in AD tangles. The presence of these bodies in the hippocampus and cortex of some patients with FTD has led to the clinical term "Pick's disease," and this term is sometimes used clinically as a synonym for various FTDs that actually have a quite diverse set of pathologies. A new term utilized to describe these disorders is "Pick complex," representing several clinical presentations with various histopathologies, including:

- Dementia with Pick bodies (or classic Pick's disease)
- Basophilic inclusion body disease (or generalized Pick's disease)
- Progressive subcortical gliosis
- Corticobasal-ganglionic degeneration
- Dementia lacking distinctive histology
- Dementia with ubiquitinated tau-negative non-eosinophilic inclusions.

In early stages, the FTDs can be difficult to diagnose and are frequently confused with psychiatric presentations. The use of positron emission tomography or single photon emission computer tomography scans may be helpful because there is frequently dramatic frontal or frontotemporal hypometabolism, even in the absence of prominent frontal or frontotemporal atrophy (**Figure 4.2** and **Color Plate 1**).

There are no therapies to prevent the progression of FTDs, and there is a clinical impression that cholinesterase inhibitors do not provide symptomatic improvement and may even increase irritability. Patients with impulsivity and compulsions may be assisted with serotonin reuptake inhibitors. Behavioral symptoms can be severe in these patients and sometimes require

FIGURE 4.2 — MRI AND PET SCANS OF A PATIENT WITH FRONTAL LOBE DEMENTIA

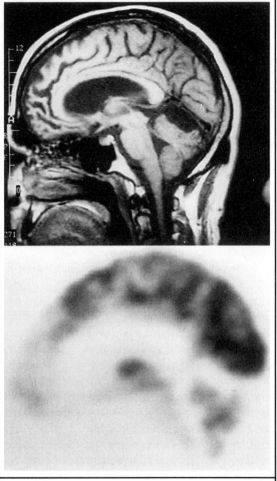

(*Top*) Magnetic resonance imaging (MRI) scan of the patient's brain, showing some frontal atrophy. (*Bottom*) Positron emission tomography (PET) scan of the same patient (same orientation), showing prominent loss of frontal metabolic activity.

multiple psychiatric hospitalizations and the use of neuroleptic and sedating medications.

Prion Diseases

Affecting humans and animals, prion diseases are an unusual group of disorders in which the infectious agent is now considered to be an abnormal conformation of a naturally occurring prion protein.[166] In humans, several of the prion diseases cause dementing syndromes, including:

- Creutzfeldt-Jakob disease (CJD)
- Gerstmann-Sträussler-Scheinker syndrome
- Fatal familial insomnia
- Kuru.

Creutzfeldt-Jakob disease is the most common of the known prion diseases with an incidence of approximately one case per million. The initial symptoms of CJD are often behavioral, with anxiety, impulsive actions, and vegetative changes, but the disease can present with cerebellar or visual problems or even with slowly progressive aphasia. A rapidly progressing dementia is characterized by personality change, agitation, paranoia, and memory deficits, leading within a few months to bedridden unresponsiveness and death. Early in the course of the disease, extrapyramidal and cerebellar signs are common. Patients may show tremor, myoclonus, exaggerated startle reflexes, seizures, lower motor neuron signs, or choreoathetotic movements.[167] Periodic sharp waves on electroencephalogram occur in a high percentage of cases, but not all. Structural imaging reveals only atrophy, although MRI with fluid-attenuated inversion recovery (FLAIR) can show increased signal in cortical or subcortical areas co-localizing with EEG abnormalities.[168] Conventional spinal fluid analysis is not helpful, however the presence of 14-3-3 protein in the cerebrospinal fluid (CSF) has been reported to have high sensitivity and specificity for CJD.[169-171]

CJD has been reported in sporadic cases and with familial pattern. Most cases of CJD occur sporadically, however, 10% to 15% of CJD cases are caused by autosomal dominant mutations in the prion protein gene, PRNP.[172] PRNP mutations can now be detected by sequencing of the prion protein gene in affected individuals and their family members, but doing so poses similar issues to testing for Huntington disease and should be approached cautiously.[173] The abnormal prion protein can also be transmitted iatrogentically.[174] Procedures involving tissue from suspected cases should always be handled carefully, since prion disease transmission has been documented to occur with:

- Corneal transplants
- Human pituitary growth hormone and gonadotropin therapies
- Dura mater grafts
- Contaminated brain electrode implants
- A variety of other neurosurgical procedures.

Cases of "classic" CJD are diagnosed in persons between the ages of 50 to 70, and these patients show dementia, myoclonus and focal signs, and very often have periodic EEG complexes. The "variant" form of CJD or vCJD, typically begins at an early age with neuropsychiatric symptoms and sensory symptoms, and these patients do not show periodic EEG complexes.[175,176] The causative agent in vCJD appears to be the same as that in bovine spongiform encephalopathy (BSE), and all confirmed cases of vCJD have come from the United Kingdom following an outbreak of BSE among cattle there, presumably as a result of eating beef from infected animals.

Huntington's Disease

This autosomal dominantly inherited disorder is characterized by chorea, neuropsychiatric symptoms, and dementia. The cognitive and psychiatric features of Huntington's disease (HD), which may precede the chorea by years, include:

- Deficits in attention, executive function and immediate memory with relative sparing of language[177]
- Personality changes and conduct disorders
- Depression, anxiety, or psychosis.

Huntington's disease can be diagnosed by demonstration of an expanded number of repeats of a polymorphic CAG sequence on the short arm of chromosome 4.[178,179] Definitive presymptomatic screening for HD is available, and ethical guidelines that should accompany such testing have been suggested. Extensive counseling, neurologic and psychologic assessment, and post-test support have been considered essential elements in the presymptomatic screening for HD.[180] Treatment revolves around management of the psychiatric symptoms and the movement disorder. New strategies that may provide symptomatic relief, restoration of function, or neuroprotection are in development or in clinical trials.[181]

Dementia Associated With Human Immunodeficiency Virus Infection

Human immunodeficiency virus-infected patients are vulnerable to a host of opportunistic infections of the central nervous system (CNS). However, direct HIV infection of the CNS is estimated to cause cognitive impairment in 20% to 30% of patients with advanced HIV disease,[182] and in 50% of acquired immunodeficiency syndrome (AIDS) patients who come to autopsy.[183,184] The pathophysiology of HIV dementia appears to involve damage from toxic viral proteins or "virotoxins" that are released from infected glial cells.[185,186] HIV dementia[187] presents initially with:

- Poor concentration
- Forgetfulness
- Depression and apathy
- Weakness and incoordination
- Myoclonus.

Caused by a latent JC polyomavirus, progressive multifocal leukoencephalopathy (PML) is a subacute, progressive, demyelinating disease of the CNS that develops in about 4% of HIV-positive patients as well as other patients who are immunosuppressed. Patients with PML typically have cognitive impairment, headache, hemiparesis, visual-field abnormalities, and coordination and gait difficulties. Computed tomography and MRI show multiple, often confluent, nonenhancing white-matter lesions. A positive JC-virus polymerase chain reaction (PCR) from CSF is specific for the diagnosis of PML; however, a negative PCR does not exclude the diagnosis.[188]

Other relatively common neurologic problems associated with HIV include varicella encephalitis and an atypical lymphoma.

Treatment of patients with HIV-related dementias depends upon the underlying etiology.

5 Risk Factors, Genetics, Biomarkers, and Diagnostic Accuracy

Factors That Increase and Decrease Risk

In epidemiologic studies, the terms "risk factor" and "protective factor" should be interpreted cautiously since the observed risk or benefit can actually be due to known or unknown confounders. The following factors have been consistently associated with greater or lesser risk of Alzheimer's disease (AD):

- *Age* is the most dramatic factor associated with increased risk of both dementia and AD (**Figure 2.1**).

- *Family history of dementia*, increases relative risk 3- to 4-fold (at least up to age 80) and is associated with total lifetime risk of 23.4% to 48.8%.[189-191] An important figure for clinicians to know when they are asked by a family member about his or her own risk is this: The cumulative incidence of AD in first-degree relatives of individuals with AD is 41% by the ninth decade of life for White Americans with even higher risks for dementia in African Americans (**Figure 5.1**).[189,191] Curves for describing the lifetime risk associated with being a first-degree relative of a patient with AD are now available for clinicians who wish to counsel family members about their own risk of developing AD.[191,192]

- *Genetic factors,* including both deterministic mutations and susceptibility genes, can alter the

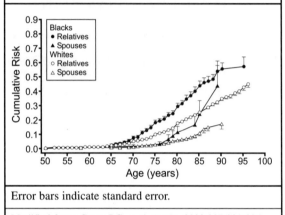

FIGURE 5.1 — CUMULATIVE RISK OF DEMENTIA IN FIRST-DEGREE BIOLOGICAL RELATIVES AND IN SPOUSES OF AD PATIENTS, STRATIFIED BY ETHNICITY OF AD PATIENTS

Error bars indicate standard error.

Modified from: Green RC, et al. *JAMA*. 2002;287:329-336.

risk of AD.[10,193] The genetic factors associated with AD are described further below.

- *Female gender* confers a slightly greater risk for AD in some studies, but not all, whereas men are at a somewhat greater risk for vascular dementia (VaD). The additional risk associated with female gender may be particularly strong among women with the apolipoprotein E (APOE) ε4 allele.[194]

- *Education* is a protective factor against dementia in a number of epidemiologic studies,[195] with a risk ratio of about 2 in favor of those with higher education. The association of dementia/AD with low education may be explained by the concept of "neurologic reserve." Thus the brain of someone who can achieve advanced education is more likely to have a higher number of neurons or synapses such that their symptoms appear relatively later, and this neurologic reserve may allow them to resist disease onset or progression for a longer period of time.

- *Head injury* is a consistent risk factor for AD,[196] an association supported by the finding of diffuse β-amyloid–containing plaques similar to those in AD in the brains of boxers with dementia pugilistica.[197] Individuals with the APOE ε4 allele (see below) may be relatively more vulnerable to poor cognitive outcome after head injury than those without this allele.[198,199]

- *Vascular disease* is a cause of dementia in its own right, so it is difficult to tease apart the degree to which vascular risk factors or cerebrovascular disease may contribute to the risk of AD. However, stroke itself may be associated with later AD among older individuals.[200] Moreover, there is evidence that among those who come to autopsy and have brain pathology of AD, the symptomatic expression of the disease may be much more severe in those who have also experienced even small cerebral infarctions.[113] Vascular risk factors have been implicated not only in VaD, but independently as risk factors for AD as well, but this is a confusing area of research. There are mixed findings about the effects of smoking,[201,202] coronary artery disease,[203-205] and hypertension.[206,207] Diabetes appears to be a risk factor for AD,[208-210] but mixed evidence generally suggests that elevated lipids and cholesterol are not risk factors for AD.[211,212] Cognitive decline has been described following coronary artery bypass grafting procedures.[213-215] In some studies, it appears to be transient,[215] while in others it appears to have long-term impact,[216] and it remains unclear whether this is a risk factor for later AD.

Other Possible Risk and Protective Factors

There are conflicting reports suggesting that other factors may influence the risk of AD, but these are less well established. For example, some data support the notion that mental inactivity in midlife is associated with an increased risk of AD,[217,218] which have led some to suggest that "mental exercise" can fend off the disease, but these findings may instead reflect the impact of very early subclinical disease. There is some evidence that midlife depression,[219,220] or even a proneness to psychological distress,[221] can increase subsequent risk of developing AD.

Increased physical activity such as walking has been reported to preserve cognitive function and reduce the risk of dementia.[222,223] Diets that are high in antioxidants, red wine, and even olive oil have been implicated as possibly protective against AD,[224-226] and moderate amounts of alcohol may be protective.[227] Some epidemiological studies suggest that diets lower in calories and fats,[228] or higher in fish or n-3 fatty acids,[229] may lower the risk of AD, but prospective trials have not been done. Elevated levels of plasma homocysteine have been associated with increased risk of AD in some studies[230] but not others,[231] and trials are underway to examine the impact of multivitamin supplementation with subsequent reduction of plasma homocysteine, on patients with AD. Risk and protective factors associated with specific medications are summarized in Chapter 8, *Current and Emerging Therapies*.

The Genetics of Alzheimer's Disease

Alzheimer's disease has an important genetic component.[10,232,233] Even before the identification of specific genes, this was clear because:

- AD occurs more commonly in families of patients with AD[191]
- AD dementia and neuropathology are associated with trisomy of chromosome 21 (Down syndrome)
- In rare families with specific mutations, AD segregates as an autosomal dominant trait over multiple generations (**Figure 5.2**).

There is some confusion about the use of the term "familial Alzheimer's disease" (FAD), since AD is a common disease and there will frequently be two or more relatives in a family who have had a dementing illness. FAD is often used loosely to describe the condition in such families, but this term should probably be reserved for the illness in families in which several members show the disease phenotype, often at an early age, and with a segregation pattern that suggests autosomal dominant inheritance (**Figure 5.2**). FAD is usually clinically and histologically indistinguishable from the typical forms except for the earlier age of onset in some pedigrees. Deterministic AD mutations have been identified in three regions:
- The amyloid precursor protein gene
- The presenilin (PS-1) gene, which codes for a transmembrane protein
- A second presenilin (PS-2) gene, which also codes for a transmembrane protein.

These genes have been identified and mapped (**Figure 5.3**), although additional mutations causing autosomal dominant patterns of inheritance are likely.[234] In some families, the PS1 mutation is accompanied by a spastic paraparesis.[235] Families with autosomal dominant FAD are of great scientific interest, but these families are quite rare, constituting less than 5% of the families who have AD. Such a family should

5

FIGURE 5.2 — FAMILIAL ALZHEIMER'S DISEASE PEDIGREE

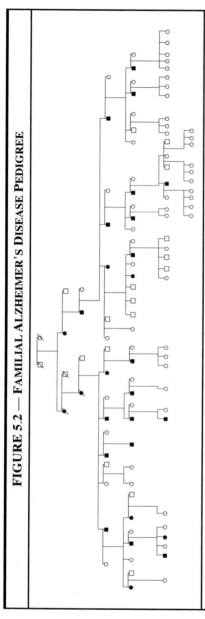

This pedigree shows the affected (solid symbols) and unaffected (open symbols) individuals across several generations in a family with the presenilin (PS-1) mutation for Alzheimer's disease.

FIGURE 5.3 — KNOWN MUTATIONS AND POLYMORPHISMS ASSOCIATED WITH AD

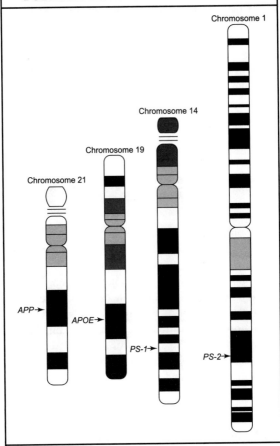

Ideograms of human chromosomes 21, 19, 14, and 1 showing the cytogenetic locations of the genes for amyloid precursor protein (APP), apolipoprotein E (APOE), presenilin-1 (PS-1), and presenilin-2 (PS-2). Mutations of APP, PS-1, and PS-2 are deterministic, whereas the presence of the ε4 allele increases susceptibility to Alzheimer's disease (AD).

Lendon CL, et al. *JAMA*. 1997;277:826.

be suspected where there is very early onset AD (in the third, fourth, or fifth decades) or when there is a family history suggestive of autosomal dominant inheritance. Genetic testing, either for diagnosis or predictive purposes, can be offered.[165] Genetic analysis of more typical cases of AD suggests that multiple susceptibility genes "mix and match" with known and unknown environmental risk factors to determine whether and when a particular individual will develop AD.[10,232] The most well-established of these susceptibility genes in AD are the polymorphisms associated with the ApoE protein.

Apolipoprotein E and Alzheimer's Disease

Apolipoprotein E is a plasma protein synthesized by the liver and also produced by astrocytes, Schwann cells, and oligodendrites in the central nervous system. It transports cholesterol and lipids between cells, is involved in the building and reinnervation of neuronal cells following injury, and may be associated with the production or deposition of amyloid, the binding of tau, and the pathophysiology of AD.[236-240] The gene (APOE) that codes for the ApoE protein has 3 alleles, designated ε2, ε3, and ε4. The inheritance of the ε4 allele is a powerful risk factor for AD in analyses of both patient populations and collections of brain-bank tissue.[241-243] The presence of the ε4 allele is not only associated with an increased chance of ultimately developing AD but is also associated with an earlier age of disease onset.[244] However, the observation that roughly 50% of the late-onset AD patients have no ε4 makes it clear that other factors are involved in the pathogenesis of the disease. The association of the ε4 allele with AD has been confirmed in many studies, but strength of this association appears to vary in different ethnic groups.[193] The presence of the ε4 allele also appears to be a strong clinical predictor of progression from mild cognitive impairment (MCI) to outright dementia.[245]

In comparison to the most common combination (ε3/ε3), the presence of a single ε4 allele triples the risk of having AD, whereas the presence of two ε4 alleles increases that risk by about 15-fold.[193] The ε4 allele is the most robust risk marker for AD currently known, probably accounting for about half of the genetic risk in the disease.

Under some circumstances, APOE genotyping may be helpful in the diagnostic workup of demented patients (see below)[246] but is currently not recommended for predictive risk assessment except within highly controlled research environments such as the Risk Evaluation and Education in Alzheimer's (REVEAL) Study.[247] Funded by the National Institutes of Health, the REVEAL Study is a research project currently under way to offer nondemented adult children of parents with AD estimates of their own risk of developing AD, including disclosure of their APOE genotype. (For further information, call 1-888-458-BUAD.) Thus far, the REVEAL Study has developed genotype-specific risk curves,[191,192] explored why first-degree relatives choose to obtain APOE testing for risk assessment,[248-250] and described the emotional and behavioral impact of these disclosures.[251-253]

Other Genetic Markers for Alzheimer's Disease

There is a vigorous search currently underway for additional genetic markers with complicated results that are beyond the scope of this manual. Positive associations with some polymorphisms have been reported, but have not been consistently verified by others.[254-257]

Diagnostic Accuracy and the Use of Biomarkers for Alzheimer's Disease

The diagnostic accuracy of most tests or procedures involves a trade-off between *sensitivity* (ie, the proportion of persons with the disease who are accurately diagnosed as having the disease) and *specificity* (ie, the proportion of persons without the disease who are accurately diagnosed as *not* having the disease). The health consequences and economic costs of making false-positive or false-negative diagnostic errors will dictate whether higher sensitivity, higher specificity, or high values for both are required for a test or procedure to be clinically useful. The overall utility of a test depends not only on sensitivity and specificity but also on the prevalence of disease in the setting where the test is intended to be used. The sequential use of any additional diagnostic test or procedure that has a positive association with the disease will always lower the sensitivity and raise the specificity. Thus when evaluating the accuracy of diagnostic procedures and tests, the question becomes one of whether the increase in specificity justifies the reduction in sensitivity.

The gold standard for determining the etiology of dementia in an individual patient is still histopathologic examination of the brain. However, the diagnosis of AD can be made in life with excellent sensitivity (between 80% and 100%) in most specialized centers,[258-261] even in very mild individuals.[262] Criteria for clinical diagnosis of AD are given in **Table 5.1**.[263]

The largest study comparing the clinical diagnosis of AD to the neuropathologic findings revealed that in specialized centers, the clinical diagnosis of AD was correct 93% of the time.[261] The specificity of the clinical diagnosis was somewhat lower at 55%, but most of the cases that were incorrectly diagnosed as AD in this study had equally irreversible degenerative dementias. Thus in the diagnosis of AD, high sensitivity may be more important than high specificity, as long as clinicians do not incorrectly diagnose and miss the opportunity to treat reversible disorders.

This reasoning becomes important in evaluating the ways that biomarkers can and cannot help with the diagnosis of AD. For example, APOE genotyping, when added to the other procedures used in the clinical evaluation of AD, decreases the overall sensitivity from 93% to 61%, while increasing the specificity from 55% to 84%.[261] And even these figures, collected in highly specialized centers on patients followed for many years to autopsy, may not be generalizable to the diagnostic scenarios facing most clinicians. Thus the use of APOE genotyping in the routine evaluation of demented patients has not proven to be helpful.[247]

These points should be kept in mind as new diagnostic tests are marketed to clinicians to assist them in the diagnosis of AD. Biomarkers for AD have been sought based on the findings of elevated tau and lower amyloid-β_{42} in the cerebrospinal fluid (CSF) of patients with AD[264-267] along with elevated neural thread protein in the CSF and possibly in the urine of patients with AD.[268-270] More recently, plasma amyloid-β_{40} and plasma amyloid-β_{42} levels have been noted to increase with age, and in some studies are elevated before and during the early states of AD, but decline thereafter, and are as yet neither sensitive nor specific.[271,272] Other studies have tried to link CSF tau and CSF amyloid-β_{42} levels to detect early AD or even MCI.[273] While all of these associations are intriguing and of important scientific value in exploring the pathophysiology of AD, their value as diagnostic adjuncts to the clinical evaluation remains unproved until the appropriate validation studies are performed.

5

TABLE 5.1 — NINCDS-ADRDA CRITERIA FOR THE CLINICAL DIAGNOSIS OF AD

Probable AD
- Criteria for clinical diagnosis of probable AD:
  - Dementia established by clinical examination, documented by mental status testing, and confirmed by neuropsychologic tests
  - Deficits in two or more areas of cognition
  - Progressive worsening of memory and other cognitive functions
  - No disturbance of consciousness
  - Onset between ages 40 and 90
  - Absence of systemic or other brain diseases that could account for dementia
- Diagnosis of probable AD is supported by:
  - Progressive deterioration of specific cognitive functions such as language (aphasia), motor skills (apraxia), and perception (agnosia)
  - Impaired activities of daily living and altered patterns of behavior
  - Family history of similar disorders, particularly if confirmed neuropathologically
  - Laboratory results of:
    - Normal lumbar puncture as evaluated by standard techniques
    - Normal pattern or nonspecific changes in EEG, such as increased slow-wave activity
    - Evidence of progressive cerebral atrophy on CT by serial observation
- Features consistent with diagnosis of probable AD:
  - Plateaus in the course of progression of the illness
  - Associated symptoms of depression, insomnia, incontinence, delusions, illusions, hallucinations, catastrophic verbal, emotional, or physical outbursts, sexual disorders, and weight loss
  - Other neurologic abnormalities, especially with more advanced disease and including motor signs such as increased muscle tone, myoclonus, or gait disorder
  - Seizures in advanced disease
  - CT normal for age

- Features that make diagnosis of probable AD unlikely:
  - Sudden onset
  - Focal neurologic findings
  - Seizures or gait disturbances early in the course of the illness

Possible AD
- Criteria for clinical diagnosis of possible AD:
  - Atypical onset, presentation, or clinical course of dementia in the absence of other neurologic, psychiatric, or systemic causes
  - Presence of a second systemic or brain disorder sufficient to produce dementia but not considered to be the cause of the dementia
  - Single, gradually progressive, severe cognitive deficit identified in the absence of other identifiable cause

Definite AD
- Criteria for diagnosis of definite AD:
  - Clinical criteria for probable AD
  - Histopathologic evidence obtained from a biopsy or autopsy

Abbreviations: AD, Alzheimer's disease; CT, computed tomography; EEG, electroencephalogram

Modified from: McKhann G, et al. *Neurology.* 1984;34:939-944.

Other biomarkers have been proposed, including measurements of dystrophic neurites in olfactory epithelium,[274] biochemical abnormalities in fibroblasts,[275,276] abnormalities in platelet membrane fluidity,[277,278] and elevation in iron-binding protein P97 in blood of AD patients compared with control subjects.[279] Alteration of amyloid precursor protein (APP) forms ratio has been described in platelets as a possible biomarker of the disease and of conversion from MCI to AD.[280-282] To date, these reports offer insights into the pathophysiology of AD, but none of these tests has been sufficiently accurate or sufficiently well validated for clinical use.

While the concept of "biomarkers" generally implies a genetic or biochemical marker, there is increasing interest in structural and function imaging as a way of examining early and even preclinical disease.[283] Total brain volume, ventricular volume, entorhinal cortex volume and hippocampal volume have all been demonstrated to change with clinical progression of AD, with some studies suggesting that entorhinal cortex atrophy begins in the preclinical state, then spreads to the hippocampus as the disease progresses.[66,284-289] A new initiative from the National Institute on Aging, in conjunction with pharmacological and biotech companies, is sponsoring the Alzheimer's Disease Neuroimaging Initiative to examine the possibility of using structural or functional imaging in future treatment trials (see http://www.nih.gov/news/pr/oct2004/nia-13.htm). It has been suggested that combinations of CSF biomarkers in conjunction with clinical examination and neuroimaging studies could sharpen the diagnostic accuracy in MCI and early dementia.[290]

The current availability of biochemical or genetic markers that may *predict* the likelihood of developing AD in asymptomatic persons raises important ethical dilemmas. Unlike the testing available for Huntington's disease (HD), predictive testing using APOE genotyping is currently only capable of generating estimated risks that could provide falsely discouraging or encouraging information to individuals. The possibility that more accurate predictive testing for AD could soon be developed will only solve some of these ethical problems, since such a test may provide no information on the age of onset and therefore would be of limited value in terms of life planning.

Without an available treatment to slow the progression of AD, the clinical value of predictive information is not clear, and such information could even be psychologically destructive, as has been demonstrated in predictive testing for HD. However, as treatments are developed that can slow the progression of AD,[291] tests that can presymptomatically recognize biochemical or genetic markers, and tests that can provide early detection and diagnosis of mildly symptomatic patients will become more and more clinically relevant. As genetic information provides a more fully refined window into the future health status of individuals, we will need to face thorny ethical issues involving the impact of such information upon those who are tested, the rights of individuals to learn such predictive information, and the retention of confidentiality of such information.[292-295]

6 Natural History

As the population ages and our society faces a greater prevalence of Alzheimer's disease (AD), clinicians who see older patients will be more involved with the care of demented patients at every stage of its course, from mildest symptoms (or even pre-symptomatic prevention) to death. Families will expect disease management information about the natural course of the disease, including projections of decline and disability, to help anticipate problems or plan for clinical and support services.

The issues associated with management of a patient who is living independently with only mild impairment are different from those associated with an end-stage patient in the nursing home. However, the principles remain the same. For every patient at every stage of the disease, the clinician's goal should be to help the patient, family, or care facility preserve the patient's independence and quality of life, while protecting the patient (and others in society) from harm.

Rate of Progression in Alzheimer's Disease

One of the most common questions that a family member (or sometimes a patient) will ask is "How fast will this progress?" At first, answering this question is difficult, since there is no *in vivo* measure of neuronal degeneration associated with AD. Sometimes the rate of disease progression can be estimated by sequential testing with neuropsychologic scales, at least in the early stages. The rate of clinical deterioration usually progresses most slowly during the earliest stages of the disease, then accelerates as the disease becomes more severe (**Figure 6.1** and **Figure 10.1**).[296,297]

FIGURE 6.1 — TYPICAL VARIATIONS IN THE COURSE OF AD DECLINE: GRAPH OF MINI-MENTAL STATE EXAMINATION SCORES

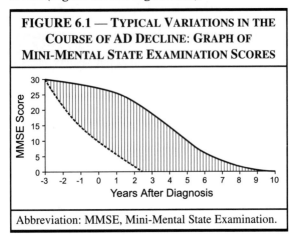

Abbreviation: MMSE, Mini-Mental State Examination.

Rate of progression in AD appears to be faster in the presence of extrapyramidal symptoms (EPS) or in the presence of psychotic or agitated symptoms, including early sleep disturbances.[298-303] Patients with pronounced aphasia, apraxia, or agnosia may also decline more rapidly.[304] It is not entirely clear whether symptom progression in AD is related to familial aggregation.[305]

There is long-standing interest in whether patients in whom the onset of AD occurs at an early age (earlier than age 60) are clinically or pathologically different from patients whose symptoms begin later. There is some evidence that the former decline more rapidly,[306,307] but others disagree,[297,302,308-312] and it may be that the disease simply appears to progress more rapidly in younger victims because of the contrast between societal expectations of younger and older individuals. AD patients who have early onset of symptoms do have more severe attentional and language deficits than patients whose symptoms begin at a later age.[311,313-315] However, there do not appear to be pathophysiologic differences between patients with early- and late-onset disease.

Clinical Heterogeneity in Alzheimer's Disease

While classic AD progresses in most patients with a fairly predictable course that begins with difficulties in new learning, the symptoms of AD may occasionally begin with isolated deficits in language, visuospatial abilities, or executive functions.[316-323] The clinical diagnosis in these cases is usually less certain. For example, the syndrome of primary (or slowly) progressive aphasia is a specific language deterioration without involvement of other cognitive domains.[324,325] Some cases of slowly progressive aphasia have been followed for years without developing significant amnesia[326] and, at autopsy, have revealed spongiform degeneration rather than AD.[327] Other patients who initially seemed to have a slowly progressive aphasia eventually became more globally demented and were found to be clinically and pathologically similar to routine cases of AD[319,328,329] or to have Pick-variant pathology.[330] A number of cases of slowly progressive apraxia have been described with neuropathologically verified AD.[88,318,331-335] While some patients with AD progress more rapidly than expected, others progress slowly and can show remarkable stability of either selected cognitive domains or even of overall intellectual function over time.[336,337]

Extrapyramidal symptoms are common in AD, occurring in at least one third of AD patients by the time they are severely impaired, even in the absence of neuroleptic medications.[338-341] AD patients with EPS may be particularly vulnerable to drug-induced parkinsonism, and when EPS occur, they are generally characterized by rigidity and bradykinesia, while tremor is rare. Many, but not all, patients with EPS who come to autopsy have pathologic changes of Parkinson's disease or Lewy body disease,[299,342] and AD patients with EPS may have a more rapid progression of cognitive symptoms, more depression, a higher rate of mortality, and a worse behavioral prognosis as the disease progresses.[339,343-345] Mild EPS and release phenomena are often noted in normally aging persons where they are associated with an increased risk of developing AD,[346-348] but these signs are considered too subtle and too infrequent to serve as diagnostic markers.[349] However, EPS, release phenomena, and pyramidal signs (extensor plantar reflexes, hyperactive jaw jerk) become more prevalent with functional impairment in severe AD.[350]

Myoclonus is often considered a late sign in AD, but rarely it may actually be associated with early onset and more rapid intellectual deterioration.[340] Although the mechanism of myoclonus in AD is not clear, it may occur through reduced sensitivity of the remaining muscarinic receptors.[351]

Clinicopathologic correlation has suggested that in patients with autopsy-proven AD, cogwheel rigidity is associated with loss of pigmented neurons in the substantia nigra and the presence of Lewy bodies in the brain-stem and cortex, and myoclonus is associated with lower neuronal counts in the dorsal raphe nucleus and locus caeruleus.[352]

Normal Aging and Mild Cognitive Impairment

There continue to be debates about how cognition changes as we age in the absence of disease and the exact nature of normal cognitive aging. However, it is now clear that much of the cognitive decline previously attributed to age alone actually reflects the effect of mild unrecognized dementia. Studies of optimally healthy older adults who are evaluated each year suggest that overall cognitive function may slow somewhat but does not decline appreciably with age, at least until the ninth decade. Therefore, in the absence of dementia or other diseases, older adults can expect stable overall cognitive function and little or no interference with performance of everyday activity[353,354] This requires a fundamental shift in the approach to the aging patient, in that clinicians should no longer automatically attribute memory or cognitive problems that interfere with everyday activities to normal aging.

Among adults over 85 years of age, the definitions of "normal" cognition are much more difficult to establish. Many neuropsychological tests have not been validated in this group of the "oldest old", and vision and hearing problems often interfere with examinations of neuropsychological domains. Nonetheless, unimpaired individuals over 85 are at high risk of developing cognitive decline, particularly those who have poorer memory or at least one APOE ε4 allele.[354]

Older patients commonly complain of memory or concentration problems, but memory complaints in the absence of discernible memory difficulties do not appear to be good predictors of current cognitive impairment[355,356] or of future cognitive impairment;[312,357] and they may be better markers of depression. On the other hand, there are a number of studies that suggest that poor performance on verbal or visual memory tasks can predict who will develop AD, sometimes up to 15 years later.[358] Some older adults, both those who complain and those who do not, may be functioning quite well in their daily life and do not meet clinical criteria for a dementing illness, yet show mild impairments with cognitive testing on a single domain, such as memory. This category of patients are now being described as having mild cognitive impairment (MCI).[134,359,360]

Mild Cognitive Impairment

MCI is used to refer to people who have evidence of cognitive impairment, but do not meet clinical criteria for dementia. MCI is not yet a fully realized diagnostic entity but is currently a subject of intense investigation and competing models of characterization. While all MCI cases are not prodromal AD, almost all AD cases will go through an MCI stage. One common way to subdivide the entity of MCI is into "amnestic" and "non-amnestic" forms, that can be further subdivided into "single domain" and "multiple domain"(**Figure 6.2**).[361]

■ **Amnestic MCI**

Patients with the amnestic form of MCI may be characterized this way:

- Memory complaint or problem corroborated by an informant
- Memory impairment on mental status or psychometric testing
- Normal general cognitive function, aside from memory
- Normal activities of daily living for his/her age
- Does not meet criteria for AD or another dementing illness.

Most persons with amnestic MCI will progress to AD at a rate of approximately 15% per year, a rate that is much higher than the incidence rate in the general population.[362-369] The average time frame in which patients with MCI progress to frank dementia is 3.5 years,[370] and progression to AD is more rapid in those with poorer cognitive measures,[371] hippocampal atro-

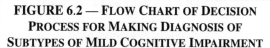

FIGURE 6.2 — FLOW CHART OF DECISION PROCESS FOR MAKING DIAGNOSIS OF SUBTYPES OF MILD COGNITIVE IMPAIRMENT

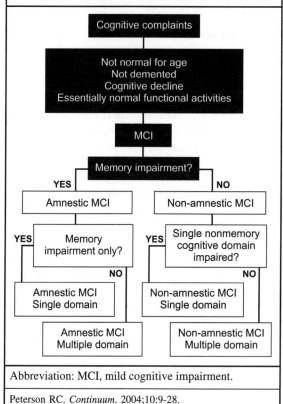

Abbreviation: MCI, mild cognitive impairment.

Peterson RC. *Continuum*. 2004;10:9-28.

phy,[284] hypoperfusion on functional scan,[372] the ε4 allele of the APOE gene,[373] or with prominent white matter changes on MR scan.[374] When there is a discrepancy between complaints of the patient and complaints of the family member, there is also more likelihood of conversion to AD.[375] When such individuals do eventually come to brain autopsy, they are most likely to have neuropathology of AD, leading many to conclude that amnestic MCI is simply an early stage of AD.[376] Amnestic MCI commonly have neuropsychiatric symptoms, particularly dysphoria, apathy, irritability, and anxiety.[377]

■ Non-Amnestic MCI

Non-amnestic forms of MCI are less well characterized, but as the name implies, have preservation of memory, along with cognitive deficits in one or more non-memory neuropsychological domains. Although some patients who meet this description will also go on to AD, the diagnoses of dementia with Lewy bodies, frontotemporal dementias and vascular dementias will be much more likely in this category.[361]

While the syndrome of MCI has not yet emerged as a diagnostic classification, consensus guidelines for approaching this area have been created,[359] and patients with MCI can be differentiated and enrolled in clinical trials.[378] Several major treatment trials designed to slow progression of memory deficits in persons with MCI have been completed or are currently under way and are discussed more fully in Chapter 8, *Current and Emerging Therapies*.

Early or Mild Alzheimer's Disease

One of the characteristics of patients with mild AD is the preservation of social and conversational skills. To the casual observer, these patients often appear completely normal in conversation. Because of this, and because some clinicians do not routinely test for mental status in older individuals, mild AD is often unrecognized, and memory complaints from a patient or family that are not associated with severe functional impairment may be dismissed or minimized. When this happens, the opportunity is lost to recognize mild AD and to provide early education and treatment. While there are many variations and some patients present atypically, the classic presentation of early AD involves:

- Impaired ability to learn and remember recently learned material
- Additional impairment in at least one other cognitive domain such as:
  - Attention
  - Problem solving
  - Language
  - Visuospatial function
  - Praxis
- Increased passivity and diminished spontaneity.

Some patients develop awareness of these symptoms, and along with these symptoms, depression may add to their cognitive difficulties. Behavioral problems are generally not seen in the earliest stages of typical AD. Formal criteria for the clinical diagnosis of AD are presented in **Table 5.1**.

Because the most characteristic cognitive feature in AD is an early and progressive deficit in the consolidation of new information into memory, simple tests of delayed word-list recall may be useful in screening for MCI or mild cases of AD. The commonly held impression that AD patients are able to recall long past events better than more recent ones is only superficially true. These patients have, in fact, been shown to recall public events inaccurately regardless of whether they occurred in recent or remote decades.

Moderate Alzheimer's Disease

As AD progresses, symptoms in other areas besides memory become more obvious. These include language problems and word-finding difficulties, along with the cognitive impairments in the domains described above. Behavioral problems, psychiatric symptoms, and agitation often appear. Family members and business associates are drawn into the patient's daily life, serving as surrogates to the patient's failing memory.

Motoric functions, such as balance and gait, are largely preserved (in the absence of EPS), but in the moderate-to-late stages of the disease, visuospatial deficits and apraxias combine to interfere with even simple activities of daily living, such as walking, dressing, and eating.

Advanced Alzheimer's Disease

The management of patients with severe AD has received less attention, but is no less important to the family, or as a situation requiring humane and thoughtful care.[379] As memory and language deficits worsen, patients may have significant word-finding and comprehension difficulties, becoming incomprehensible and, ultimately, even mute. Eventually, they deteriorate to a stage of complete helplessness with inability to speak, eat, or even move. Mortality is higher among those patients with a more rapid rate of clinical decline.[380] In clinical practice, we have the impression that death occurs about 8 to 10 years after diagnosis or a bit earlier in patients with hypertension, wandering, falling, and behavioral problems. However, the median survival in all patients may be shorter than this.[381] In the severe stages of the disease, death usually occurs from respiratory infection.

Since there is no agreed upon standard for the treatment of complications in late-stage dementia, there are considerable clinical, ethical, and health policy problems associated with using aggressive medical interventions.[382] Providing palliative care at home, in a nursing home, or in a hospice setting can spare patients invasive diagnostic workups, is associated with lower observed discomfort, and may aid the family with the grieving process.[383]

7

Pathophysiology and Neuropathology

The cause of Alzheimer's disease (AD) is not yet fully understood, but clues from genetics, pathology, biochemistry, and a variety of basic sciences are rapidly converging to increase our understanding of the pathophysiology and provide new opportunities for treatment. However, it is clear that AD is a complex disease, in that it has both genetic and environmental precipitants, and that as a result of the disease, the affected brain endures structural changes and alterations in neurotransmitter systems.

Pathophysiology and Neuropathology of Alzheimer's Disease

Grossly, AD accentuates the changes in brain weight, volume, ventricular size, and gyral atrophy that occur with normal aging. The frontal and temporal lobes are more involved than other regions, and the hippocampus is often atrophic.[384,385] There are numerous neuropathologic changes in the brain of patients with AD, but the major histopathologic hallmarks of AD are:

- Neurofibrillary tangles (NFTs)
- Amyloid-beta (Aβ) peptide deposition in senile plaques (SPs) and blood vessels
- Neuronal death.

Neurofibrillary tangles are masses of abnormal filaments within the cytoplasm of neurons that are made up of paired helical filaments.[386-388] The major protein abnormality in NFTs is the presence of a highly insoluble, hyperphosphorylated microtubule-associated protein called tau.[389] The intracellular deposition of tau and its disruption of the normal cytoskeletal architecture may be an important factor in the death of neurons.[390] Some researchers believe that treatments directed toward inhibiting NFTs may be helpful in treating AD.[391]

Amyloid deposition appears to play a critical role in the pathophysiology of AD.[392-394] The amyloid precursor protein (APP) molecule is a transmembrane protein of unknown function. In humans, the predominant metabolism of APP involves an enzyme, termed the α secretase, that cuts the extracellular portion of the molecule at a site close to the membrane surface, producing a long protein comprised entirely of the extracellular portion of the molecule. This portion of the molecule is known as soluble APP α.

In AD, as demonstrated most clearly in the mutations that cause dominantly inherited familial forms, this normal metabolism is altered (**Figure 7.1**). The APP molecule is cut at a different, extracellular site by one enzyme (termed the β secretase) and again within the transmembrane region by another enzyme (called the γ secretase).[395] One of the molecular fragments produced by these cuts is either 40 or 42-43 amino acids in length, and this fragment is termed the Aβ or β-amyloid fragment. In AD, the alternative cleavage pattern of APP and the resulting production of β-amyloid are increased, resulting in the deposition of β-amyloid in SPs and blood vessels.

The amyloid hypothesis as the proximate cause of cell death in AD is supported by considerable evidence. β-amyloid production is increased in APP and presenilin mutations that cause AD, and in transgenic mice that exhibit AD phenotypes. Accumulation of β-amyloid is toxic to neurons in cell culture, and is increased in the presence of the APOE ϵ4 allele. Nevertheless, there are challenges to the amyloid hypoth-

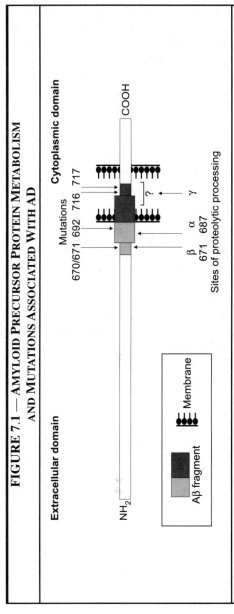

FIGURE 7.1 — AMYLOID PRECURSOR PROTEIN METABOLISM AND MUTATIONS ASSOCIATED WITH AD

Diagram of the amyloid precursor protein (APP) showing the location of the familial Alzheimer's disease-causing mutations (codons 670/671, 692, 716, 717) and the sites of proteolytic cleavage (α-, β-, γ-secretase cleavage sites). Aβ indicates β-amyloid fragment.

esis in that the correlation between amyloid deposi-
tions and dementia is not robust. Other hypotheses
emphasize neurofibrillary pathology,[391] or that β-amyloid toxicity may depend upon soluble oligomers of
β-amyloid termed Aβ-derived diffusible ligands
(ADDLs).[396,397] There are probably distinctive stages
in the initiation and progression of AD pathology such
that deposition of β-amyloid reaches a "ceiling' early
in the disease process, while NFT formation, synaptic
loss and gliosis continues throughout the disease.[398]
Thus, it makes sense that in many studies, NFT counts
and cell loss are more associated with cognitive decline than amyloid burden.[399]

Senile plaques are spherical structures averaging
about 100 microns in diameter, composed of degenerating neuronal processes, extracellular Aβ, microglia, and astrocytes.[400-402] The *neuritic* plaques (NP),
with abnormal neuronal processes surrounding an amyloid core, are distinguished from the *diffuse* plaques
(DP), which are amorphous amyloid deposits without
dystrophic neurites (**Figure 7.2**). Aβ is deposited in
NP and in the walls of the cerebral vasculature in all
AD cases. The initial Aβ deposition in AD appears to
involve $Aβ_{1-42}$, which is present in both DPs and NPs.
Deposition of $Aβ_{1-40}$ occurs predominantly in NPs and
blood vessels.[393]

Neuronal death occurs in normal aging, but patients with AD lose more neurons than normal at an
earlier age. Cell death in the brain occurs through a
combination of factors that is sometimes loosely described as apoptosis or programmed cell death, and in
AD, the effects of phosphorylated tau or Aβ deposition may accelerate this process. Another mechanism
that may accelerate cell death is inflammation of the
brain of patients with AD, especially in the region of
the NP.[403,404] For example, deposition of Aβ may initiate an inflammatory response through the activation

FIGURE 7.2 — CLASSIC PATHOLOGY OF AD

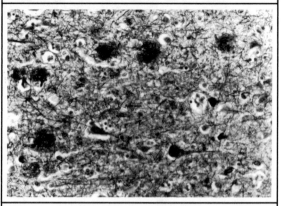

The neurofibrillary tangles (elongated dark objects) and neuritic plaques (larger, round, dark objects) are the classic neuropathologic finding in the brain of patients with Alzheimer's disease (AD).

7

of the receptor for advanced glycation end products, leading to a subsequent cascade of increasingly cytotoxic events, such as free radical formation, oxidative stress, disturbance of calcium homeostasis, and mitochondrial membrane disruption **Figure 7.3**.[405-407] Antioxidant and anti-inflammatory treatments are therefore under consideration for patients with AD (Chapter 8, *Current and Emerging Therapies*).

Neurotransmitter System Abnormalities

Neurotransmitter system abnormalities in AD have attracted considerable attention for their relevance to potential pharmacologic interventions. The discovery that cortically projecting cholinergic cells in the basal forebrain's nucleus basalis of Meynert are devastated in AD[408,409] and the subsequent replications and exten-

FIGURE 7.3 — INFLAMMATORY CASCADE

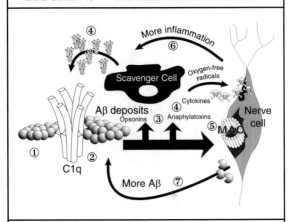

Inflammation and Alzheimer's disease (AD). 1) Most of the inflammatory mechanisms in the AD brain is believed to be responses to neurodegeneration and to amyloid β (Aβ) peptide. 2) Complement component C1q, for example, binds Aβ and the classical complement pathway is activated. 3) Complement opsonins and anaphylatoxins recruit and activate microglia, the brain's resident scavenger cell. 4) Activated microglia produce more complement, as well as reactive oxygen species and proinflammatory cytokines. 5) Complement activation also results in formation of the membrane attack complex (MAC), which can lyse neurons. 6) All of these mechanisms feed back to fuel more inflammation. 7) Some inflammatory mediators have also been implicated in Aβ production and aggregation into plaques.

Diagram courtesy of Dr Joe Rogers.

sions of these observations have contributed to the notion of this disease as a cholinergic dementia.[410] The activity of choline acetyltransferase (ChAT), the enzyme responsible for the synthesis of acetylcholine (ACh), is markedly reduced in the cortices of AD patients when compared with age-matched controls.[408,411]

Enthusiasm for a cholinergic interpretation of AD has inspired many attempts to treat AD with cholinergic drugs, as summarized in Chapter 8, *Current and Emerging Therapies*. The cholinergic synapse consists of presynaptic and postsynaptic portions (**Figure 7.4**). In the presynaptic portion of the synapse, ACh is synthesized by ChAT from choline and acetyl coenzyme A. Following its release at the synapse, ACh is rapidly degraded by the enzyme acetylcholinesterase. Within the synapse, there are postsynaptic (M1) receptors and presynaptic (M2) autoreceptors. The postsynaptic receptors are relatively preserved providing an opportunity for stimulating the cholinergic neurotrans-

FIGURE 7.4 — THE CHOLINERGIC SYNAPSE

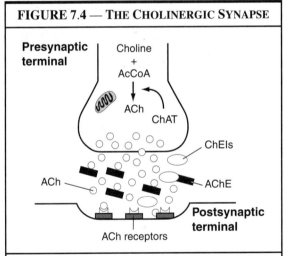

The cholinergic synapse consists of presynaptic and postsynaptic portions. In the presynaptic portion of the synapse, acetylcholine (ACh) is synthesized by choline acetyltransferase (ChAT) from choline and acetyl coenzyme A (AcCoA). Following its release at the synapse, ACh is rapidly degraded by the enzymes acetylcholinesterase (AChE). Cholinesterase inhibitors (ChEIs) block the action of the AChE enzyme, allowing ACh to remain active longer within the synaptic cleft.

mitter system. Strategies to enhance the cholinergic system have included dietary choline, muscarinic receptor agonists to stimulate M1 receptors, and cholinesterase inhibitors to slow ACh degradation (Chapter 8, *Current and Emerging Therapies*).

However, cholinergic deficits in AD are not the exclusive neurochemical deficit. Neurochemical deficiencies occur among almost all neurotransmitter types.[412] For example, noradrenergic neurons are depleted in the locus coeruleus,[413-416] and there is a significant decrease in tyrosine hydroxylase, the rate-limiting enzyme for norepinephrine synthesis.[417] Neurons in the dorsal raphe nucleus are also lost in AD, and levels of both serotonin and 5-hydroxyindoleacetic acid are diminished.[415,418] Alterations in other neurotransmitters, including glutamate and glutamic acid decarboxylase/γ-aminobutyric acid have also been reported.[419-422] A variety of neuropeptide abnormalities also have been documented in AD. Prominent among these are reductions in somatostatin, neuropeptide Y, and vasopressin.[423]

Indeed, any amyloid-bearing NP in the cortex of patients with AD may contain degenerating neurites of varying neurotransmitter specificities, including substance P, somatostatin, neurotensin, cholecystokinin, leucine enkephalin, and vasoactive intestinal polypeptide.[424] Similarly, although many cortical NFTs display cholinesterase activity,[425] tangles are seen in serotonergic-, noradrenergic-, and somatostatin-reactive neurons in AD.[415,426]

Criteria for Neuropathologic Diagnosis of Alzheimer's Disease

From a clinician's viewpoint, the histopathologic examination of the brain by an experienced neuropathologist is the gold standard for diagnosis. Thus it sometimes comes as a surprise to learn that the criteria for making the diagnosis of AD neuropathologically have been debated and revised in recent decades.

The plaques and tangles originally observed in the brains of AD patients by Alois Alzheimer in 1911 were never obvious to pathologists who only used standard staining techniques (such as hematoxylin and eosin) because these features are best seen with silver stains or special stains such as thioflavine-S. Neuropathologic criteria for the diagnosis of AD were first standardized by consensus in the 1980s to require specific age-defined neocortical densities of SPs and NFTs.[427] These criteria required the presence of SPs and NFTs in the neocortex in numbers >2 to 5 per microscope field of 1 mm^2 for persons younger than age 50; >8 per field, with some tangles permitted for persons aged 50 to 65; >10 per field, again with some tangles in persons aged 66 to 75; and plaques numbering >15 per field in persons over 75, though neocortical tangles were not required.

The use of these criteria[428] or similar SP and NFT counts[429] for the diagnosis of AD resulted in fairly good interrater reliability among academic neuropathologists. However, these criteria were variably applied by practicing neuropathologists,[430] perhaps because the criteria were less accurate in older individuals with milder cognitive changes.[431,432] Moreover, a number of additional problems were recognized with these criteria:

- The type of SP was not specified
- Quantification of SPs was difficult
- The presence of NFTs was required only for the youngest cases
- Important areas of allocortex were not formally included in the evaluation, and the relationship to clinical history was vague.[433]

In 1991, the Consortium to Establish a Registry for Alzheimer's Disease (CERAD) proposed semi-quantitative criteria emphasizing NP in three neocortical regions: middle frontal gyrus, superior/middle temporal gyri, and inferior parietal lobule.[434,435] Once again, the criteria were age-dependent (younger than 50, 50 to 75, over 75, respectively) to take into account the confounding age effect in using NPs to diagnose AD. This information was integrated with the clinical history to achieve a definite, probable, or possible diagnosis of AD. In summary, the CERAD criteria placed considerable emphasis on NPs, did not emphasize NFTs or important allocortical regions, and the semiquantitative approach was somewhat subjective.[433] Nonetheless, the CERAD criteria gained wide acceptance.

Subsequently, a 6-tier system based upon the distribution pattern of NFTs and neuropil threads was proposed for staging changes in AD.[436,437] These criteria do not emphasize NPs and are not specific about the quantification of neurofibrillary pathology. Preliminary reports have partially validated these criteria,[438] but further clinicopathologic correlation studies are needed, especially in the oldest old.

The most recently developed criteria arose from the Workshop on Diagnostic Criteria for the Neuropathological Assessment of Alzheimer's Disease. These criteria include major changes to previous approaches as follows:

- Elimination of the previous NIA-NINCDS (Khachaturian) criteria
- Use of semiquantitation of NP as in the CERAD criteria and elimination of diffuse plaques for diagnosis
- Addition of semiquantitation of neocortical NFTs

- Additional examination of the hippocampus and entorhinal cortex
- Emphasis on defining coexisting pathologic lesions.[439]

Animal Models of Alzheimer's Disease

Alzheimer's disease does not occur in animals, and there are no perfect animal models. Recently, the development of transgenic mice has provided models that are intriguing.[440-442] For example, mice with a mutant APP gene expressing transforming growth factor β-1 develop amyloid plaques more quickly than the transgenic mice without that gene.[443] Similarly, doubly transgenic mice expressing familial AD-linked variants of both presenilin-1 and APP show evidence of amyloid deposition at a younger age than mice expressing only mutant APP.[444,445] Further, when transgenic mice that overexpress a human APP mutation and develop large deposits of Aβ are crossed with apolipoprotein E (APOE) "knockout" mice (which are missing the gene for APOE), the amount of Aβ deposited in the brains of the progeny is markedly decreased, suggesting a major role for APOE in the formation of amyloid deposits and new directions for therapy.[446] In the future, various types of genetically altered "designer" mice will likely play an important role in understanding of the pathophysiology of AD and developing new treatments.

7

8   Current and Emerging Therapies

Managing Alzheimer's Disease

Alzheimer's disease (AD) is a family-systems disease, causing tremendous upheaval and morbidity for the patient and for everyone in the patient's family. At every stage of the disease, the patient's deterioration requires increasing resources. At every stage of the disease, the family requires new information and access to new services. Typically, families look to their primary medical clinician to be their interpreter and referral source—someone to prioritize and guide them through the maze of issues they may be facing for the first time (see Chapter 11, *Resources for Clinicians and Families*).

While it is exciting to have new and effective pharmacologic treatments for AD, clinicians who make the diagnosis of AD and dispense prescriptions without additional effort do their patients a great disservice. Education and family support efforts are critical aspects of the appropriate management of patients with AD and their families, and have been demonstrated to reduce caregiver burden and morbidity and even to delay nursing-home placement.[447] Even if families do not immediately process the educational efforts or use the referral services at the time they are provided, they may still benefit from them later. Therefore, at the time that the diagnosis of AD is made or in subsequent appointments over the following weeks, every patient/family in whom AD is diagnosed should receive:

- An explanation of the diagnostic process and the disease itself (see Chapter 3, *Evaluation of*

113

the Older Patient With Cognitive Problems,
Chapter 7, *Pathophysiology and Neuropathology*, and Chapter 10, *Family Education and Support*)

- A general description of the prognosis and what to expect in terms of cognitive decline, possible behavioral symptoms, and increasing levels of dependency (see Chapter 6, *Natural History,* and Chapter 9, *Management of Agitation and Behavioral Symptoms*)
- An overview of available pharmacologic treatments, including their medical benefits, financial costs, and possible side effects (this chapter) and a treatment recommendation
- Inquiries and preparations about the burdens of caregiving (see Chapter 10, *Family Education and Support*)
- Referral to the local Alzheimer's Association for further education and caregiver support and introduction to educational materials (see Chapter 11, *Resources for Clinicians and Families*)
- Information about local social workers and lawyers specializing in the management of elders with cognitive impairment (see Chapter 10, *Family Education and Support*).

Pharmacologic Therapy for Alzheimer's Disease

Pharmacologic therapies are an exciting and rapidly changing component of the management strategy for AD. Distinctions should be made between therapies that provide proven symptomatic improvements, such as the cholinesterase inhibitors (ChEIs) and *N*-methyl-D-aspartate (NMDA) receptor antagonists (**Figure 8.1**, *left*) and disease-modifying therapies that may prevent the onset or slow the progression of the disease, such as antioxidant treatments (**Figure 8.1**, *right*).

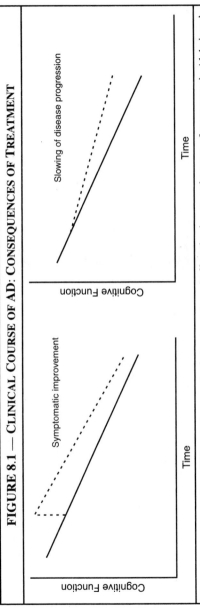

FIGURE 8.1 — CLINICAL COURSE OF AD: CONSEQUENCES OF TREATMENT

Symptomatic improvement

Cognitive Function

Time

Slowing of disease progression

Cognitive Function

Time

These figures suggest how different pharmacologic treatments may affect the downward course of symptoms in Alzheimer's disease (AD) and show the distinction between a treatment that improves symptoms and one that slows disease progression. The cholinesterase inhibitors have been shown to provide symptomatic improvement but not to modify disease progression. As of this writing, no compounds have been definitively shown to slow disease progression, although there is preliminary experimental evidence for vitamin E, as well as observational evidence for estrogen replacement and anti-inflammatory compounds.

With some compounds, (anti-inflammatory agents and hormone replacement therapies [HRTs]), there have been separate trials to explore the possibility of both symptomatic and disease-modifying properties.

The distinction between symptomatic and disease-modifying treatments is frequently misunderstood by both clinicians and families, leading to unrealistic expectations. Since every medication choice weighs the anticipated benefits against the side effects and financial costs of that therapy, it is particularly important that clinicians inform patients accurately. Providing accurate information on the anticipated benefits, side effects, and cost is a key step in the treatment protocol for the use of pharmacologic therapies in AD.

Overview of Treatment Strategies for Alzheimer's Disease

The categories of potential pharmacologic strategies for AD now and in the near future are summarized in **Table 8.1**.[448] The following categories of therapy are discussed below:
- Cholinergic enhancement
- NMDA receptor antagonism
- Antioxidant treatment
- Anti-inflammatory treatment
- Hormone therapies
- Other therapies.

Although new clinical evidence is being continuously generated, as of this publication date, only the ChEIs and one NMDA receptor antagonist have been demonstrated to have therapeutic efficacy with acceptable side effects in multiple, large-scale, randomized clinical trials. Several other types of symptomatic and disease-modifying treatments have shown promise and are currently undergoing clinical trials.

TABLE 8.1 — POTENTIAL PHARMACOLOGIC APPROACHES TO THERAPY FOR AD

Cholinergic Enhancements
- Acetylcholine precursors
- Acetylcholine agonists
- Cholinesterase inhibitors
- Growth factors

N-methyl-D-aspartate Receptor Antagonism
- Memantine

Other Neurotransmitter System Modifications
- Serotonin agonists or reuptake inhibitors
- Corticotropin-releasing factor enhancers
- Thyrotropin-releasing hormone and analogues
- Prolyl endopeptidase inhibitors

Antioxidants and Vitamins
- Vitamins C and E
- Monoamine oxidase type B inhibitors
- Coenzyme Q
- Propentofylline

Anti-inflammatory Agents
- Glucocorticoids
- Nonsteroidal anti-inflammatory drugs
- Cyclooxygenase-2 inhibitors

Hormone Therapies
- Estrogen
- Selective estrogen receptor modulators (SERMs)
- Anti-luteinizing hormone therapies

Other Potential Therapies

This table summarizes recent pharmacologic approaches to the treatment and/or prevention of Alzheimer's disease (AD). While clinical trials are under way or planned for many of the treatments above, only the cholinesterase inhibitors and memantine have been demonstrated to be efficacious in multiple, large-scale clinical trials.

Cholinergic Enhancement

Many years prior to the recognition of cholinergic deficits in AD patients, drugs such as scopolamine that block acetylcholine (ACh) receptors were noted to produce transient impairments of cognitive function and memory that were reversible with physostigmine, an acetylcholinesterase inhibitor.[449,450] Later, as described in Chapter 6, *Natural History*, the loss of cholinergic neurons in the basal forebrain and the corresponding loss of cortical cholinergic projections were strongly associated with memory deficits and other cognitive impairments in AD. In particular, deficits in choline acetyltransferase, a key enzyme in the synthetic pathway for ACh, have been consistently noted in the neocortex of patients dying with AD, along with the relative preservation of muscarinic postsynaptic receptors.[408-410,412,451-458]

For many years after this, the most intensive focus for treatment studies in AD were attempts to supplement cholinergic function, at first through dietary supplements, and later through direct-acting agonists or ChEIs. In the 1980s, treatment trials with oral choline or lecithin (precursors to ACh), with direct-acting agonists and with intravenous or oral physostigmine, sometimes in combination with dietary ACh precursors, did not demonstrate encouraging efficacy. ChEIs were also considered for treatment in the hope that inhibiting the hydrolysis of ACh in the synaptic cleft would effectively increase the amount of ACh available for cholinergic receptors. In theory, this would partly counteract the cholinergic insufficiency associated with AD neuropathology.

■ Cholinergic Agonists

The theoretical benefit of cholinergic receptor agonists is based upon the fact that postsynaptic muscarinic (M_1) cholinergic receptors are relatively intact in AD, while presynaptic (M_2) receptors, which regulate ACh release, are decreased.[454] Moreover, muscarinic agonists may also alter amyloid precursor protein (APP) processing and reduce amyloid-β protein secretion.[459] Prior trials of bethanechol and arecoline have shown minimum efficacy and substantial side effects. Newer, more specific agents that have been evaluated clinically include xanomeline, milameline, memric, and others, but trials thus far have not demonstrated greater efficacy or markedly better side-effect profiles than the ChEIs.[460-462] The potential role of nicotinic agonists in the treatment of AD is unclear and no large-scale clinical trials evaluating these compounds have been reported to date.

■ **Cholinesterase Inhibitors**

Hydrolysis of synaptic ACh can occur either by specific central nervous system acetylcholinesterases (AChEs) or by nonspecific cholinesterases, such as butylcholinesterase, that are located in both the central and peripheral nervous systems (**Table 8.2**). ChEIs that can cross the blood-brain barrier will delay the intrasynaptic degradation of ACh, presumably prolonging its effects. The principal side effects of ChEIs are due to the enhancement of cholinergic activity in the gastrointestinal (GI) tract, therefore more specific agents will have fewer GI side effects.

Cholinesterase-inhibiting drugs can be grouped into three broad classes based on structure and mode of inhibition:

- Tertiary and quaternary amines, which are reversibly inhibitory; they exhibit both competitive and noncompetitive inhibition, which is short-term and directly dependent on drug concentration.
- Organophosphates, which form an extremely stable enzyme-inhibitor complex, resulting in irreversible inhibition; onset of inhibition is

TABLE 8.2 — SECOND-GENERATION CHOLINESTERASE INHIBITORS AVAILABLE FOR AD

Generic (Trade) Drug Name	Enzyme Interaction	AChE Selectivity	Plasma $t_{\frac{1}{2}}$ (h)	Recommended Starting (Maximum) Dosage/d (mg)	Hepato-toxicity
Donepezil (Aricept)	Reversible	Selective	70-80	5 qd (10)	No
Galantamine (Reminyl)	Reversible	Selective	Short	4 bid (32)	No
Rivastigmine (Exelon)	Reversible	Selective	2*	1.5 bid (12)	No

Abbreviation: AChE, acetylcholinesterase; AD, Alzheimer's disease.

* The duration of actual cholinesterase effect is days to weeks.

Modified from: Schneider LS, Tariot PN. *Med Clin North Am.* 1994;78:911-934 and Farlow MR, Hake AM. *Int J Geriatr Psychopharmcol.* 1998;1:S2-S6.

rapid (minutes) and duration is longer than 6 hours.

- Carbamate inhibitors, which are pseudo-irreversible. By mimicking ACh, they form a covalently bound carbamoylated complex that inactivates AChE temporarily until the carbamate moiety is replaced by a hydroxyl group (about 10 hours).

■ Clinical Use of Cholinesterase Inhibitors

In 1986, the oral administration of tetrahydroaminoacridine (tacrine), a centrally active ChEI, demonstrated modest, dose-related improvements in performance-based tests in large-scale clinical trials (**Table 8.3**).[463-465] The Food and Drug Administration (FDA) approved tacrine in 1993 for use in AD, despite the clinical trial results showing modest efficacy, a frequent dosing schedule, and a high prevalence of GI side effects, along with the need to monitor liver function studies for potential hepatotoxicity.[466-468] Nevertheless, the efficacy of tacrine in some patients was unequivocal, and it represented a first step toward the treatment of a previously untreatable disease.[469,470]

The development and approval of tacrine helped to create a consensus among industry, academic, and government experts on standards for dementia trials. In particular, a standard for dual efficacy in clinical trials of symptomatic treatments for AD has emerged in which the FDA requires evidence of improvement on a measure of cognitive performance as well as on a scale of caregiver/clinician assessment. The most common primary outcome measures in each of these categories that have been utilized in recent clinical trials are the performance-based Alzheimer's Disease Assessment Scale-Cognitive Subscale (ADAS-Cog) and the semi-structured Clinician's Interview-Based Impression of Change with caregiver input (CIBIC-Plus), respectively. The ADAS-Cog is a multi-item in-

8

TABLE 8.3 — LARGE, RANDOMIZED, PLACEBO-CONTROLLED TRIALS OF CHOLINESTERASE INHIBITORS AND NMDA RECEPTOR ANTAGONISTS IN PATIENTS WITH AD

Study	Duration (weeks)	MMSE Scores of Patients Enrolled	Daily Dose (mg)	Number of Subjects Enrolled	Improvement Over Placebo on ADAS-Cog With ITT Analysis	Attrition (%)	Attrition Due to Side Effects (%)
Tacrine (Farlow, 1992[a])	12	10-26	Placebo	77		27	Not published
			20	158	NS	38	
			40	156	NS	47	
			80	37	2.8	52	
Tacrine (Knapp, 1994[b])	30	10-26	Placebo	181		33	Not published
			40/80	80	1.4	40	
			40/80/120	174	2.0	70	
			40/80/120/160	263	2.2	73	
Donepezil (Rogers, 1996[c])	12	10-26	Placebo	40		13	5
			1	42	1.6	19	12
			3	40	2.1	5	5
			5	39	3.2	13	8

Donepezil (Rogers, 1998[d])	12	10-26	Placebo 5 10	150 156 155	 2.5 3.1	7 10 18	2 4 10
Donepezil (Rogers, 1998[e])	24	10-26	Placebo 5 10	153 152 150	 2.5 2.9	20 15 32	7 6 16
Rivastigmine (Corey-Bloom, 1998[f])	26	10-26	Placebo 1-4 6-12	235 233 231	 2.1 3.8	17 15 35	7 8 29
Rivastigmine (Schneider, 1998[g])	26	10-26	Placebo 3 6 9	173 175 177 177	Not published	Not published	Not published
Rivastigmine (Rosler, 1999[h])	26	10-26	Placebo 1-4 6-12	239 243 243	 1.6 1.6	13 14 34	7 7 23

Continued

8

Study	Duration (weeks)	MMSE Scores of Patients Enrolled	Daily Dose (mg)	Number of Subjects Enrolled	Improvement Over Placebo on ADAS-Cog With ITT Analysis	Attrition (%)	Attrition Due to Side Effects (%)
Galantamine (Raskind, 2000[i])	24	11-24	Placebo 24 32	213 212 211	 3.9 3.4	19 32 42	8 23 32
Galantamine (Tariot, 2000[j])	21	10-22	Placebo 8 16 24	286 140 279 273	 1.3 3.1 3.1	16 23 22 22	7 6 7 10
Memantine (Reisberg, 2003[k])	28	3-14	Placebo 20	126 126	6.1*	33 23	17 10
Memantine (Tariot, 2004[l])	24	5-14	Placebo† 20	201 203	3.4*	25 15	12 7

Abbreviations: ADAS-Cog, Alzheimer's Disease Assessment Scale-Cognitive Subscale [scores]; ITT, intent-to-treat; MMSE, Mini-Mental State Examination; NMDA, N-methyl-D-aspartate; NS, not significant.

* These studies of more severely impaired patients did not use the ADAS-Cog, so change scores on the Severe Impairment Battery (SIB) are shown. SIB scores are not directly comparable to ADAS-Cog scores.

† In this study, all patients were receiving stable doses of donepezil before and throughout the trial.

[a]Farlow M, et al. *JAMA.* 1992;268:2523-2529; [b]Knapp MI, et al. *JAMA.* 1994;271:985-991; [c]Rogers SL, Friedhoff LT. *Dementia.* 1996;7:293-303; [d]Rogers SL, et al. *Arch Intern Med.* 1998;158:1021-1031; [e]Rogers SL, et al. *Neurology.* 1998;50:136-145; [f]Corey-Bloom J, et al. *Int J Geriatr Psychopharmacol.* 1998;1:55-65; [g]Schneider LS, et al. *Int J Geriatr Psychopharm.* 1998;1:S26-S34; [h]Rosler M, et al. *BMJ.* 1999;318:633-638; [i]Raskind MA, et al. *Neurology.* 2000;54:2261-2268; [j]Tariot PN, et al. *Neurology.* 2000;54:2269-2276; [k]Reisberg B, et al. *N Engl J Med.* 2003;348:1333-1341; [l]Tariot PN, et al. *JAMA.* 2004;291:317-324.

8

strument examining memory, orientation, attention, reasoning, language, and praxis (scored between 0 and 70) that has been well validated in longitudinal cohorts of AD patients.[471-474] The CIBIC-Plus is a semi-structured interview that utilizes both caregiver and clinician perceptions to rate the degree of global improvement or deterioration from one visit to the next, with scores ranging from 1 (marked improvement) through 4 (no change) to 7 (marked worsening).[475,476] Secondary outcome measures that have been gathered in clinical trials of symptomatic treatment for AD include additional measures of cognitive performance (such as the Mini-Mental State Examination [MMSE]), measures of behavioral symptoms (see Chapter 9, *Management of Agitation and Behavioral Symptoms*), and numerous scales of functional abilities and caregiver burden. The American Academy of Neurology currently recommends that treatment with ChEI "should be considered" in anyone with a diagnosis of AD.[133] The average cost of ChEI treatment is $1200 to $1800 per year, however, most pharmacoeconomic studies suggest that if initiated early, and continued for at least 2 years, the cost of ChEI treatment can be recouped by savings through reduced care costs and delayed nursing home placement.[477]

Comprehensive review of treatment trials and recommendations for ChEI can be found elsewhere,[133,477] and highlights of these and other studies are summarized below.

Tacrine

Tacrine (tetrahydroaminoacridine) (Cognex), an acridine-based reversible, nonspecific ChEI, was the first ChEI approved for the therapy of AD as described above. Tacrine is considered a first-generation ChEI because it is relatively nonselective, and thus a high prevalence of GI side effects (ie, nausea, vomiting, diarrhea, and cramping) limit the tolerability of the agent.

Tacrine induced elevated liver function tests (primarily serum aminotransferase) in up to 40% of patients and required serum monitoring of liver function tests. With the availability of more selective second-generation ChEIs, treatment of patients with tacrine is no longer recommended.

Donepezil

Donepezil (Aricept) is a second-generation, highly selective piperidine-based ChEI with a long plasma half-life (70 to 80 hours) and elimination through both renal excretion of intact drug and biotransformation via the cytochrome (CYP) P450 system. Dosage adjustment is not necessary in patients with renal or hepatic disease. There is no evidence of significant drug-drug interactions.

Large-scale, double-blind, placebo-controlled trials with donepezil in patients with mild-to-moderate AD (MMSE 10 to 26) have demonstrated significant improvements in cognition, global functioning, and activities of daily living (**Figure 8.2** and **Table 8.3**).[478-480] One year placebo-controlled trials demonstrated that donepezil is effective for at least this period of time[481] and could delay the loss of some functional measures by 5 months.[482] And donepezil has been shown to be associated with lower levels of behavioral disturbances[483] and to improve cognition, behavior, and activities of daily living, as well as reduce caregiver burden, in more severely impaired AD patients (MMSE 5-17).[484,485] Donepezil has been reported to improve cognition in vascular dementia (VaD)[132,486] and in the dementia of Parkinson's disease.[487,488]

Donepezil is currently indicated for the treatment of mild-to-moderate AD and has been used extensively in clinical practice throughout the world. Dosages of both 5 mg/day and 10 mg/day are effective with trends toward greater efficacy at the higher dose (**Figure 8.2**). In practice, the higher dose is associated with a higher

8

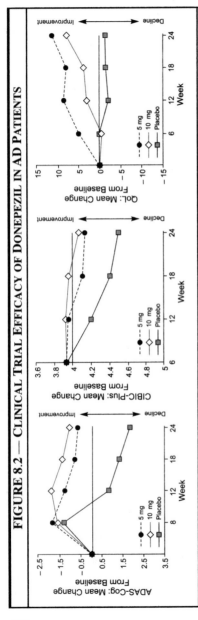

FIGURE 8.2 — CLINICAL TRIAL EFFICACY OF DONEPEZIL IN AD PATIENTS

These figures demonstrate the results of one trial of donepezil in patients with mild to moderately severe Alzheimer's disease (AD). Outcome measures are the Alzheimer's Disease Assessment Scale-Cognitive Subscale (ADAS-Cog), the Clinician's Interview-Based Impression of Change Plus (CIBIC-Plus), and the Quality of Life Scale (QoL). The results of this and other trials are summarized in **Table 8.3**.

Rogers SL, et al. *Neurology*. 1998;50:136-145.

incidence of cholinergic side effects, particularly GI symptoms. Titration should be slow, and patients should be on a 5-mg dose for 4 to 6 weeks before raising the dose to 10 mg.

In a 24-week randomized controlled trial of 270 patients with mild cognitive impairment (MCI), the group treated with donepezil did not show significant differences on the primary outcome measures but the patients on donepezil did better on some secondary measures and, of course, had more side effects.[489] A preliminary report of a large 3-year randomized trial of patients with MCI has suggested that on average, those treated with donepezil progressed to AD 6 months later than those randomized to placebo.[490] However, the difference between the treated and untreated groups, which was seen at 18 months, was no longer apparent by the end of 3 years.

Rivastigmine

Rivastigmine (Exelon) is a second-generation, highly selective carbamate ChEI. Rivastigmine binds to AChE and dissociates slowly, providing a reversible AChE inhibition that lasts much longer (10 hours) than its plasma half-life of 1 to 2 hours. Because of rivastigmine's rapid hydrolysis to the decarbamoylated metabolite, both *in vitro* and animal studies have shown major CYP P450 isoenzymes to be minimally involved in the drug's metabolism. No pharmacokinetic drug interactions with drugs metabolized by the CYP enzyme systems were expected or seen in clinical trials.[491] Renal elimination is rapid and complete.

Large-scale, double-blind, placebo-controlled trials with rivastigmine in patients with mild-to-moderate AD (MMSE 10 to 26) have demonstrated significant dose-dependent improvements in cognition, global functioning, and activities of daily living (**Figure 8.3** and **Table 8.3**).[492,493] Rivastigmine has also been shown to improve behavioral symptoms in AD.

FIGURE 8.3 — CLINICAL TRIAL EFFICACY OF RIVASTIGMINE IN AD PATIENTS

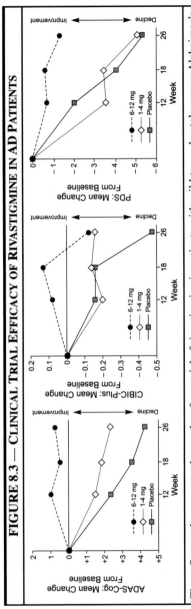

These figures demonstrate the results of one trial of rivastigmine in patients with mild to moderately severe Alzheimer's disease (AD). Outcome measures are the Alzheimer's Disease Assessment Scale-Cognitive Subscale (ADAS-Cog), the Clinician's Interview-Based Impression of Change Plus (CIBIC-Plus), and the Progressive Deterioration Scale (PDS). The results of this and other trials are summarized in **Table 8.3**.

Corey-Bloom J, et al. *Int J Geriatr Psychopharmacol.* 1998;1:55-65.

Rivastigmine is currently indicated for the treatment of mild-to-moderate AD after having been evaluated in clinical trials involving over 3300 patients worldwide. Clinical efficacy was evaluated both at low doses (1 mg to 4 mg daily) and high doses (6 mg to 12 mg daily), with clear evidence of better efficacy at the higher dose range (**Table 8.3**). The higher dose is associated with a higher incidence of cholinergic side effects, particularly GI symptoms. Titration should be slow, and patients should be on a low dose for 4 to 6 weeks before increasing to a higher dose. Efficacy has been demonstrated even in AD patients with concurrent vascular risk factors.[494]

Galantamine

Galantamine (Reminyl) is a second-generation, selective and reversible ChEI. Galantamine, a tertiary alkaloid with a dual mechanism of action, is also an allosteric modulator of presynaptic and postsynaptic nicotinic receptors. Galantamine is well absorbed, although food delays the distribution of drug, and it has a terminal elimination half-life of about 7 hours. Plasma protein binding is low. Galantamine is metabolized by CYP 450 enzymes and excreted in the urine, and inhibitors of CYP2D6 and CYP3A4 can modestly increase the bioavailability of the drug. Patients with hepatic or renal disease should be treated cautiously.

Large-scale, double-blind, placebo-controlled trials with galantamine in patients with mild-to-moderate AD (MMSE 10 to 24) and have demonstrated significant improvements in cognition, global functioning, and activities of daily living,[495-497] as well as improvement in behavioral symptoms (**Figure 8.4**).[496] The doses reported in these trials were 8 mg, 16 mg, 24 mg, and 32 mg daily, dosed according to a bid regimen. In one of these trials, significant improvement in behavioral symptoms was also noted.[496] In a trial of VaD patients who were combined with VaD patients,

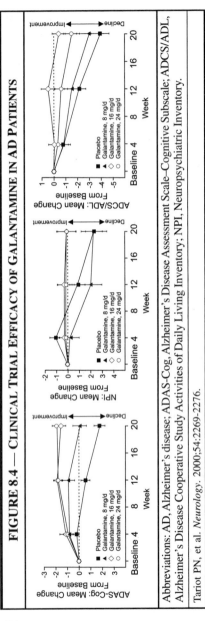

FIGURE 8.4 — CLINICAL TRIAL EFFICACY OF GALANTAMINE IN AD PATIENTS

Abbreviations: AD, Alzheimer's disease; ADAS-Cog, Alzheimer's Disease Assessment Scale–Cognitive Subscale; ADCS/ADL, Alzheimer's Disease Cooperative Study Activities of Daily Living Inventory; NPI, Neuropsychiatric Inventory.

Tariot PN, et al. *Neurology.* 2000;54:2269-2276.

galantamine also showed greater efficacy than placebo on measures of cognition, activities of daily living, and behavioral symptoms.[131]

Galantamine is currently indicated for the treatment of mild-to-moderate AD, and there is again evidence of greater efficacy at higher doses (**Table 8.3**). As with the other ChEIs, cholinergic side effects, especially GI symptoms, can occur particularly at higher doses. Subgroup analysis of "advanced moderate" patients from the pivotal trials demonstrated that these patients had sustained benefits for at least a year.[498] Galantamine may be effective in patients with dementia due to Parkinson's disease.[499]

■ Other Cholinesterase Inhibitors

Metrifonate is a second-generation, nonselective organophosphate ChEI. Metrifonate itself has no AChE inhibitory activity, but it is spontaneously hydrolyzed to 2,2-dimethyl dichlorovinyl phosphate, the active compound, which inhibits AChE by stable binding to the catalytic site of the enzyme. Several large-scale, double-blind, placebo-controlled trials with metrifonate in patients with mild-to-moderate AD (MMSE 10 to 26) demonstrated dose-dependent improvements in cognition, global functioning, and activities of daily living that were roughly comparable to those seen with other ChEIs.[500] However, the manufacturer and the FDA suspended clinical trials of metrifonate after several patients experienced muscle weakness which required a period of respiratory support, and further development has been halted.

Huperzine A (HupA), a sesquiterpene alkaloid extracted from moss (Huperzia serrata), is a reversible ChEI that has been used in China for centuries for the treatment of swelling, fever, and blood disorders. It has recently been the subject of double-blind, placebo-controlled clinical trials in patients with AD, largely in China, with indications of improved cognitive function and quality of life.[501] Trials in the United States are underway.

■ Common Side Effects of Cholinesterase Inhibitors

The second-generation ChEIs are generally well tolerated and the most common side effects are mild GI problems. Since appetite may be diminished and already-frail patients may lose weight, it is useful to follow a patient's weight. While ChEIs reduce agitation (see below), occasionally patients become more agitated or experience disrupted sleep. The common side effects of ChEIs, roughly in order of frequency, are as follows:

- Nausea
- Anorexia
- Dyspepsia
- Diarrhea
- Vomiting
- Fatigue
- Dizziness
- Insomnia
- Muscle cramps
- Agitation.

■ Other Features of Cholinesterase Inhibitors

To date, no distinctive subpopulations (age, gender, APOE genotype) of patients have been identified that will show greater benefit with ChEIs than others. There is some evidence that patients who are progressing most rapidly show greatest benefit to rivastigmine.[502]

Only a few large-scale, randomized, placebo-controlled clinical trials of ChEIs have lasted more than 30 weeks. When treatment is discontinued in most ChEI trials, the ADAS-Cog scores and CIBIC-Plus ratings for the treatment groups rapidly declined to levels that were not significantly different from those of the placebo group, suggesting that the beneficial ef-

134

fects of ChEIs rely upon continued administration. However, at least one combined analysis of the retrieved dropout population from several large trials with rivastigmine suggest that ChEI's may have a more lasting effect on disease progression.[503] Uncontrolled data from patients on open-label donepezil have suggested that efficacy may persist for several years,[504,505] and recent data from a large-scale, placebo-controlled trial of donepezil over 1 year indicated that treated patients were able to maintain some functional abilities 5 months longer than untreated patients over the year.[482] A large meta-analysis indicated that ChEIs can modestly improve neuropsychiatric and functional outcomes.[506]

While a number of large-scale clinical trials have shown the efficacy of the ChEIs, there have been far fewer studies that have focused upon when to begin these treatments, how to choose optimal dosing, when and how to change compounds, and how long to continue treatment.[477] However, the best evidence available and clinical experience suggests that early initiation of treatment provides greater long-term benefits, and that stopping and restarting treatment may cause loss of benefits in comparison with those who do not stop. Switching from one ChEI to another is a reasonable strategy and can be done without a washout period for those who have not responded to the first ChEI, or with a washout period of 5 to 7 days for those who had significant side effects on the first ChEI. In switching to ChEI's that recommend a titration period, the titration scheme should be followed when starting the new treatment. For suggestions on how long to continue treatment with a ChEI, see **Table 8.4**.

NMDA Receptor Antagonism

Memantine, a compound that blocks NMDA receptors, has emerged as the first noncholinergic treat-

TABLE 8.4 — TIPS FOR USING CHOLINESTERASE INHIBITORS IN PATIENTS WITH ALZHEIMER'S DISEASE

- Establish a specific diagnosis of Alzheimer's disease (AD) using clinical assessment, laboratory studies, and neuroimaging
- Assess the severity of the dementia, preferably using a staging instrument or mental status questionnaire
- Establish accurate and realistic expectations for treatment benefits, costs, and side effects
- Start treatment at low dosages and increase dosages every 3 to 6 weeks as tolerated to maximum recommended levels
- Evaluate efficacy and side effects, particularly weight loss, every 2 to 3 months for several visits
- Evaluate and manage patient agitation and caregiver distress
- Continue cholinesterase inhibitor (ChEI) therapy if there appears to be stabilization in functional, cognitive, or behavioral decline
- Well-controlled data are not available on the long-term efficacy of ChEIs after 1 year. There are two approaches to long-term continuation:
  - If side effects are not unacceptable, maintain therapy until the patient's quality of life is too impaired to justify the potential benefit or financial cost of further symptomatic treatment
  - Continue ChEI therapy as long as cognitive function is stabilized. If cognition declines, reduce the dose of the ChEI and observe for accelerating deterioration. If deterioration is accelerated, reintroduce ChEI therapy. If discontinuing treatment has no effect, ChEI therapy can be stopped
- Discontinue ChEI therapy in patients requiring general anesthesia

ment to demonstrate efficacy in AD. Clinical data on memantine is provided below. This section describes the theoretical basis of how NMDA receptor blockers may work in AD.

Glutamate is a major excitatory neurotransmitter in the brain. NMDA receptors are present on many excitatory synapses, but are not thought to contribute to synaptic excitation under normal resting conditions.[507] However, with increased synaptic excitation, the neuron sufficiently depolarizes so that the effective binding affinity for Mg^{2+} for the channel-blocking site is reduced, and NMDA receptors can be activated by synaptically released glutamate. When NMDA receptors remain open longer, they permit the entry of Ca^{2+} ions into the cell, which can then activate Ca^{2+} dependent protein kinases, leading to long-term potentiation, a form of cellular learning. However, under some pathological conditions, the neuronal membrane is chronically depolarized, leading to prolonged Ca^{2+} influx, which can then trigger a cascade of neuronal injury and cell death. Excitotoxic mechanisms such as these have been hypothesized to play a role in AD,[508] although increased glutamate levels have not been documented in the AD brain.

Competitive NMDA receptor antagonists have been logical compounds to try in a variety of neurological diseases including stroke, epilepsy, and brain trauma, without dramatic successes to date. Uncompetitive antagonists can be divided into two broad categories: dissociative anesthetic agents with high toxicity (such as PCP, ketamine and MK-801 at higher doses), and low-to-moderate affinity antagonists with a very favorable side-effect profile (such as amantadine and memantine). The theory behind treatment with low-affinity uncompetitive NMDA receptor antagonists is that blocking low, tonic levels of NMDA receptor–mediated excitation while still allowing NMDA receptor responses may provide symptomatic

8

improvement without disrupting normal cell function, as well as potential neuroprotective effects.[507]

It is also possible that NMDA receptor blockade could influence Aβ mediated toxicity. For example, there is some evidence that Aβ kills neurons through such mechanisms as oxidative stress, disruption of Ca^{2+} homeostasis and resulting excitotoxicity.[509] Inappropriately timed or sustained glutamate activation of NMDA receptors can contribute to this "weak excitotoxicity" and facilitate cell death, and memantine has been shown to protect against Aβ toxicity in a rat model.[510] Furthermore, Aβ may interact with NMDA receptors to enhance receptor-mediated excitotoxicity and increase neuronal vulnerability.[511] In addition, there is some evidence that NMDA-induced excitotoxicity can increase tau production,[512] and that tau phosphorylation might be reduced or prevented by NMDA receptor antagonists.[513,514] Finally, NMDA can accelerate the death of cholinergic neurons,[515] and NMDA receptor blockers, including memantine, can attenuate this process.[516,517]

Memantine

Memantine (Namenda) is an "uncompetitive" or channel-blocking NMDA receptor antagonist that is structurally similar to amantadine. Memantine was first synthesized in the early 1960s and was observed to have similar properties as amantadine in treating neurological diseases. It was used after 1978 in Germany as a "neurological tonic" for a variety of neurological diseases and after 1989 for the treatment of dementia. Time to maximum plasma concentration following oral administration ranges from 3 to 7 hours, and food does not have an effect on absorption. The terminal elimination half-life is 60 to 80 hours, with elimination predominantly through the urine, so dosage adjustment would be reasonable in patients with renal disease. Plasma protein binding of memantine is low, the CYP

P450 enzyme system is not involved in metabolizing the compound, and there are no significant drug-drug interactions, including interactions with ChEIs.

Large-scale, double-blind, placebo-controlled trials of memantine in patients with moderate-to-severe dementia (AD and VaD),[135,518] and moderate-to-severe AD[519] have demonstrated significant improvements in cognition, global functioning, and activities of daily living (**Table 8.3** and **Figure 8.5**). Memantine also demonstrates efficacy in mild-to-moderate VaD,[136] and provides additional efficacy to patients with moderate-to-severe AD who are already receiving stable treatment with donepezil.[520]

Memantine has a long history of extensive use in Europe. It was approved early in the United States in October 2003 and became available in January 2004 for the treatment of moderate-to-severe AD. Memantine can be taken with or without food and, in clinical trials, was not associated with any greater discontinuation of drug or any more side effects than seen in the placebo arm.[518,519] Recommended dosage is 10 mg bid after titration, gradually increasing by 5-mg increments occurring at least 1 week apart to 10 mg in the morning and 10 mg at night. Memantine can be added to donepezil without any increase in side effects[520] and is being tested in conjunction with other cholinesterases, where there is already a clinical impression that it can be used safely in conjunction with those as well.

Antioxidant Therapies, Vitamins, and Diet

In addition to the search for medications to improve the cognitive symptoms of AD, there has been an increasing interest in the identification of agents that could slow the progression of the disease. For example, neurons in patients with AD may be more susceptible to oxidative stress by virtue of increased monoamine

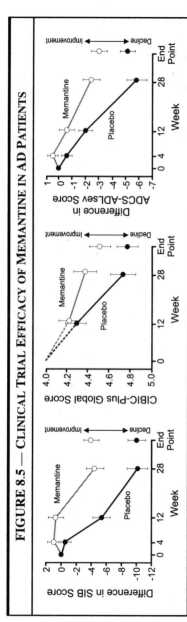

FIGURE 8.5 — CLINICAL TRIAL EFFICACY OF MEMANTINE IN AD PATIENTS

Abbreviations: AD, Alzheimer's disease; ADCS-ADLsev, Alzheimer's Disease Cooperative Study Activities of Daily Living Inventory [modified for severe dementia]; CIBIC-Plus, Clinician's Interview-Based Impression of Change Plus Caregiver Input; SIB, Severe Impairment Battery.

Reisberg B, et al. *N Eng J Med.* 2003;348:1333-1341.

oxidase (MAO) activity.[521] Free radicals, the by-products of metabolic processes such as oxidative metabolism, may accumulate, leading to excessive lipid peroxidation and neuronal degeneration in the brain. Monoamine oxidase inhibitors (MAOIs) can reduce oxidative deamination and may prevent the formation of free radicals, preserving neuronal integrity,[522] as well as produce a selective augmentation of monoaminergic transmission. Alpha-tocopherol (vitamin E), a lipid-soluble vitamin that can block lipid peroxidation, may also reduce oxidative damage.[523]

Some epidemiological studies have suggested that diets with lower calories and fats,[228] the use of antioxidant vitamin supplements[524-526] or foods rich in antioxidants[226,229] may reduce the risk of developing AD, while others have not been able to demonstrate these associations[527,528] or challenge whether retrospective studies are able to accurately measure food histories.[529] Small trials of MAOIs in patients with AD have suggested efficacy.[530] In a large 2-year, multicenter, double-blind, placebo-controlled trial, 341 patients with moderate-to-severe AD received the MAOI selegiline (Eldepryl) and alpha-tocopherol (vitamin E), either alone or in combination, or they received placebo.[531] Outcome measures were death, institutionalization, loss of ability to perform at least three activities of daily living, and severe dementia. Over the course of the 2-year trial, neither of the compounds provided cognitive improvement, but all treated groups showed less decline on an activities of daily living scale when compared with placebo. And, as shown in **Figure 8.6**, selegiline, alpha-tocopherol, or both appeared to delay progression to the mixed end point by approximately 25% over the 2 years of the study. The adjusted difference between treatment and placebo in the time to reach the first end point was 230 days for alpha-tocopherol, 215 days for selegiline, and 145 days for selegiline plus alpha-tocopherol. This study re-

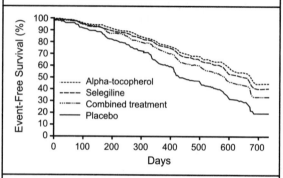

FIGURE 8.6 — SELEGILINE AND ALPHA-TOCOPHEROL (VITAMIN E) TREATMENT OF PATIENTS WITH AD

Antioxidant treatment with either selegiline or alpha-tocopherol (or both) appears to slow progression toward the end points of nursing-home placement, severe disability, or death in patients with Alzheimer's disease (AD).

Sano M, et al. *N Engl J Med.* 1997;336:1216-1222.

quired statistical adjustment to equate the initially nonequivalent treatment groups and should not be considered definitive until reproduced. However, this design signaled a new era of treatments for AD designed to slow progression or even to provide primary prevention in at-risk populations and has prompted many clinicians to treat their AD patients with daily doses of vitamin E.

For those clinicians who recommend vitamin E, the choice of dosage remains unclear. The study described above was the only large-scale treatment study, and it used 2000 IU of vitamin E daily, but this dosage can cause GI symptoms and could cause anticoagulation and bleeding problems in some patients if they have underlying liver disease. Therefore, clinicians who recommend vitamin E either for patients with AD or for those who hope that it has disease-modifying (or disease-delaying) properties, usually suggest dosages of anywhere from 800 IU to 2000 IU daily, given in 2 divided doses. The benefits of vitamin E are by no means well established, and preliminary results from a large trial examining the impact of vitamin E on slowing the transition from MCI to full dementia did not reveal any efficacy for vitamin E.[490]

Idebenone is a benzoquinone compound structurally related to coenzyme Q that not only is a long-acting ChEI but also inhibits lipid peroxidation and may function as an antioxidant or oxygen-free radical scavenger.[532] Early clinical trials suggested efficacy[533-535] but in a large 1-year randomized controlled trial of mild-to-moderate AD patients, idebenone failed to show clinically significant slowing of AD progression.[536]

The extract of the ginkgo biloba, derived from the leaves of a subtropical tree, is also believed to act as an antioxidant.[537] Several small studies[538,539] as well as two larger clinical trials[540,541] have suggested that ginkgo biloba may provide a small beneficial effect on cognitive measures in patients with AD, though others have showed no efficacy.[542] In the most highly publicized of these trials, a large number of dropouts raise questions about the validity of the results,[540] and large-scale trials to evaluate efficacy are under way. Since ginkgo biloba is sold as a health supplement, it is not subject to the same purity standards or marketing restrictions that govern FDA-approved treatments. A multicenter prevention trial using ginkgo is currently underway.

Some epidemiological studies suggest that diets lower in calories and fats[229] or higher in fish or n-3 fatty acids[543] may lower the risk of AD, but prospective trials have not been done. Elevated levels of plasma homocysteine have been associated with increased risk of AD in some studies,[230] but not others,[227] and trials are underway to examine the impact of mul-

143

tivitamin supplementation with subsequent reduction of plasma homocysteine on patients with AD.

Anti-inflammatory Therapies

As described in Chapter 7, *Pathophysiology and Neuropathology*, there is considerable evidence that immune and inflammatory reactions occur in the brain of AD patients, including the activation of complement cascades and inflammatory cytokines.[404,544] Most, [545-549] but not all,[550] epidemiologic evidence from observational studies suggest that patients exposed to long-term anti-inflammatory medications may have a reduced risk of developing AD.[551] In pilot studies, the glucocorticoid prednisone, which should suppress both acute-phase response and the complement pathway, resulted in no improvement in either behavior or cognition in 19 AD patients over a 7-week period,[552] while improvements were seen in a relatively small trial of indomethacin.[553] Among the nonsteroidal anti-inflammatory compounds, there has been considerable focus upon the cyclooxygenase (COX) inhibitors, specifically those directed at COX-2, which is activated by inflammatory stimuli.[554] However, a small trial of COX-2 inhibitors,[555] as well as well-designed 1-year trials of prednisone[556] and nonsteroidal anti-inflammatories[557] did not improve symptoms or slow decline in patients with mild-to-moderate AD. Two large trials of rofecoxib have shown that it failed to slow the progression of AD[558] or to reduce the conversion of MCI patients to dementia.[559]

The Alzheimer's Disease Anti-inflammatory Prevention Trial is a National Institutes of Health–funded project designed to determine if anti-inflammatory medications (both a general anti-inflammatory and a COX-2 inhibitor) can prevent the onset of AD in 70-year-old or older first-degree relatives of patients with

AD. (For further information, call toll-free 1-866-2-STOP-AD.)[560]

Hormone Therapies

Estrogen-sensitive neurons are present in both male and female brains and may play an important role in neurocognitive function, both in normal aging and in AD. The mechanisms through which hormones might exert these effects are varied,[561-563] but could include:

- Improved glucose transport in the hippocampus
- Promotion of neuronal viability and synaptic integrity
- Enhanced choline uptake
- Increased cerebral blood flow
- Modification of APP processing and plaque formation
- Regulation of nerve growth factor and NMDA receptors.

The term HRT encompasses estrogen replacement therapy, with and without progestins. The progestin is prescribed to prevent endometrial cancer and therefore is not necessary in women who have had a hysterectomy. SERMs are synthetic compounds that can act both as an agonist and as an antagonist at the estrogen receptor.

Interest in HRT to treat or prevent AD arose because hormone replacement was thought to improve cognition in nondemented postmenopausal women[564] and because some (but not all) observational studies have suggested that HRT in postmenopausal women with AD may be associated with improved cognition, later onset, or slower rate of progression,[565-569] although observational studies of estrogen efficacy are notoriously vulnerable to various sources of bias.[570,571] Several large clinical trials of estrogen replacement in women with or at risk for AD are under way to determine whether estrogen prevents or slows progression in women at risk for AD, and the results thus far have suggested no preventative benefit for HRT. In the Women's Health Initiative, a large randomized study comparing estrogen plus progestin to placebo, women treated with hormone therapy had *worsened* cognition,[572] and the incidence of dementia was significantly *increased* among those taking estrogen replacement (with or without progesterone), leading to the discontinuation of the study.[573,574] Two prospective trials have also shown that HRT does not provide symptomatic benefits in patients with AD.[575,576] No large-scale AD trials with SERMs have been conducted. Therefore, neither HRT nor SERMs are currently recommended for prevention or treatment of AD.

A trial of dehydroepiandrosterone (DHEA) did not demonstrate differences between treated group and placebo.[577]

Other Potential Therapies

An enormous number of strategies are under investigation for their potential as treatment or preventive agents in persons with or at risk for AD has been conducted.

Many noncholinergic neurotransmitter modifying agents to treat AD have been proposed, and tested in trials of variable size and methodologic rigor.[448,578] Opiate antagonists were at one time considered possible cognitive enhancers,[579,580] but multicenter studies failed to confirm improvement.[581,582] There have been small trials but no clear evidence of improvement in AD with ganglioside GM_1,[583] with noradrenergic replacement therapies such as clonidine[584] or guanfacine,[585] somatostatin replacement therapy with octreotide,[586] or thiamine.[587] Possible improvements have been reported in

146

trials of nicotine,[588,589] nimodipine (a calcium antagonist),[590] and acetyl-L-carnitine.[591,592] Interesting improvements in cognition have been demonstrated in AD patients after treatment with simple glucose,[593] but large-scale trials have not been conducted. A number of therapies have attempted to utilize nerve growth factor or stimulants of neurotrophic factors to preserve the viability of vulnerable cholinergic neurons, without clear benefits.[594,595] A related class of medications, the nootropics, have been widely used in Europe for years despite poor efficacy on well-controlled trials.[596-598] In the United States, a neurotrophic agent called FPF 1070 or cerebrolysin has shown mixed results in clinical trials.[599-601]

Some of the most promising therapies in development are those designed to alter the production, deposition, or clearance of amyloid-β peptide (also know as β-amyloid or Aβ).[392,393] These include the APP β and γ secretase inhibitors and the β-amyloid vaccine. Secretase inhibitors are currently in clinical trials, but no results are available as this goes to press. Both active and passive vaccination with β-amyloid proteins promotes an immune response that can reproducibly reduce amyloid burden in the brains of transgenic mice[602,603] and can reduce cognitive dysfunction in these mice.[604] An initial human trial with the Aβ vaccine AN-1792 was halted due to serious meningoencephalitic complications in some patients,[605] and there are concerns about possible toxicity of this approach.[606,607] However, the first analysis of human neuropathology from a participant in this trial who later died revealed an apparent reduction of Aβ plaques, suggesting that the strategy might be effective in humans if the problem of side effects could be controlled.[608] Analysis of a small series of patients receiving the immunization showed encouraging clinical results as well.[609] It is likely that vaccine trials will resume soon with altered compounds.[610] While most

147

new strategies for AD drug development have concentrated upon amyloid pathway, there are some compounds being explored that have the potential to impact the cascade of events leading to hyperphosphorylated tau and stabilize microtubules.[611,612]

Statins (HMG-CoA reductase inhibitors) are well-established medications that lower cholesterol and have been proven to reduce the risk of heart disease and stroke. Some case-control epidemiological studies have suggested that statins may reduce the risk of developing AD,[613-616] while several longitudinal studies have not found any protective association.[617,618] Clinical trials of statin use in patients with AD are currently underway.

Chelation therapy has been proposed for AD since metal ions (zinc, copper and iron) have been implicated in the formation of amyloid plaques. Clioquinol, a copper and zinc chelator, inhibits amyloid deposition in transgenic mouse models of AD[619] and small trials have suggested possible efficacy.[620]

Cognitive activity is frequently hailed as an antidote to cognitive decline and seniors exhorted to "use it or lose it" as if the brain were a muscle to be exercised. A number of well-designed studies have suggested that participation in leisure activities[218,621] and cognitively stimulating activities[622] can reduce the risk (or delay the development) of AD, but these findings remain difficult to interpret because subtle, manifestations of AD could reduce interest and initiative in such activities many years prior to the onset of recognizable symptoms. Nevertheless, a number of recommendations are emerging to try to maintain "cognitive vitality."[623]

Several unusual surgical treatments for AD have been piloted and are under further evaluation. These include the placement of a low-flow ventriculo-peritoneal shunt to provide chronic CSF drainage,[624] as well as omental transposition to increase cerebral blood flow to the brains.[625,626] Further trials of these procedures are underway.

As in other incurable diseases, there are frequent claims for nutritional and alternative preventatives and treatments. None of these have demonstrated efficacy but some, such as huperzine A, levacecarine, and EGB 761, warrant further investigation in controlled trials.[627]

Treatments of Normal Individuals to Prevent or Delay Onset of AD

It is well recognized that the most fruitful areas for AD treatment in the future may be compounds that prevent AD in cognitively normal persons, or slow the progression of mild cases, such as those with MCI. Despite a wealth of epidemiological evidence about compounds or lifestyle interventions that might be helpful, the trials necessary to demonstrate clear efficacy are arduous and expensive. This is a rapidly moving field, but at the time of this writing, no treatments are available that unequivocally protect normal individuals against developing AD. A number of trials are underway exploring specific compounds (**Table 8.5**).

8

TABLE 8.5 — SUMMARY OF ONGOING AND COMPLETED TRIALS EXAMINING COGNITIVE CHANGE AND INCIDENT DEMENTIA

Protocol (agents used)	N	Population	Duration	Cognitive Outcome and Result
Heart Protection Study[a] Vitamin E 600 mg Vitamin C 250 mg Beta carotene 20 mg	20,536	Men and women cardiovascular risk factors 40-80 years of age	5 years	TICSm and incident dementia No differences between vitamins and no vitamins
DATATOP[b] Selegiline 10 mg Vitamin E 2,000 IU	800	Parkinson's disease patients	2 years	Cognitive test scores No treatment differences in any cognitive measure
PREADVISE[c] Selenium 200 µg Vitamin E 400 IU	10,400	Men = 60 of age	12 years	Incident dementia and cognitive test scores Recruitment is ongoing
GEMS[d] Ginkgo biloba extract 240 mg	5,000	Men and women = 75 years of age	5 years	Incident dementia or VaD or cognitive or functional tests. Trial ongoing
HERS[e] Conjugated equine estrogen 0.625mg Medroxyprogesterone acetate 2.5 mg	1,063	Women mean age = 67 years	4.2 years	Six cognitive tests Treatment associated with lower scores on one test

WHI-PERT[f,g] Conjugated equine estrogen 0.625 mg Medroxyprogesterone acetate 2.5 mg	4,381	Women = 65 years of age	4 years	Probable dementia and 3MS scores: treatment increased risk of dementia and yielded less change in 3MS scores.
WHI-ERT Conjugated equine estrogen 0.625 mg	N/A	Women = 65 years of age		Probable dementia and 3MS scores: Recruitment complete; observation ongoing
ADAPT[h] Naproxen sodium 220 mg BID Celecoxib 200 mg BID	2,625	Family hx of AD = 70 years of age	7 years	Incident AD and cognitive tests Recruitment ongoing
Heart Protection Study[i] Simvastatin 40 mg	20,536	Men and women cardiovascular risk factors 40-80 years of age	5 years	TICSm at last visit: No difference between simvastatin vs no simvastatin
PROSPER[j] Pravastatin 40 mg/day	5,804	Men and women cardiovascular risk factors 70-82 years of age	3.2 years	MMSE, Stroop Picture word learning, letter-digit coding, Activities of Daily Living No treatment effect

Continued

8

Abbreviations: AD, Alzheimer's disease; ADAPT, Alzheimer's Disease Anti-Inflammatory Prevention Trial; DATATOP, Deprenyl and Tocopherol Antioxidative Therapy for Parkinson's Disease; GEMS, Ginkgo for the Evaluation of Memory; HERS, Heart and Estrogen/Progestin Replacement; hx, history; IU, international units; MMSE, Mini-Mental State Examination; MS, Memory Study; PREADVISE, Prevention of Alzheimer's Disease by Vitamin E and Selenium; PROSPER, Pravastatin in elderly individuals at risk of vascular disease; TICSm, modified Telephone Interview for the Cognitive Status questionnaire; VaD, vascular dementia; WHI-ERT, Women's Health Initiative-Estrogen Replacement Therapy; WHI-PERT, Women's Health Initiative-Progestin and Estrogen Replacement Therapy.

[a]Heart Protection Study Collaborative Group. Lancet. 2002;360:23-33. [b]Kieburtz K, et al. Neurology. 1994;44 :1756-1759. [c]Prevention of Alzheimer's Disease by Vitamin E and Selenium (PREADVISE). Available at: http://www.clinicaltrials.gov/show/NCT000040378. Accessed September 30, 2004. [d]Ginkgo Biloba Prevention Trial in Older Individuals, RFA: AT-99-001, National Center for Complementary and Alternative Medicine and National Institute on Aging, February 26, 1999. [e]Grady D, et al. Am J Med. 2002;113:543-548. [f]Shumaker SA, et al. JAMA. 2003;289:2651-2662. [g]Rapp SR, et al. JAMA. 2003;289:2663-2672. [h]Martin BK, et al. Control Clin Trials. 2002;23:93-99. [i]Heart Protection Study Collaborative Group. Lancet. 2002;360:7-22. [j]Shepherd J, et al. Lancet. 2002;360:1623-1630.

Sano M. CNS Spectr. 2003;8:846-853.

9

Management of Agitation and Behavioral Symptoms

Dementing disorders impair behavior and comportment (noncognitive symptoms) as well as thinking and memory (cognitive symptoms). Behavioral problems can be the presenting complaint of a dementing illness but are more often seen later in the course. Disruptive and aggressive behaviors are more stressful to family members than cognitive limitations because they cause such fatigue, embarrassment, and fear, and they are more likely to prompt institutionalization than physical infirmities or even incontinence.[628,629]

Behavioral problems become more common and more severe as cognitive abilities deteriorate, and are more common in those with at least one copy of the APOE ε4 allele.[630,631] Among community-dwelling patients 60% to 80% of those with dementia, and even 20% to 40% of those with MCI, have been reported to have multiple behavioral disturbances[632-634] In nursing-home patients, behavioral problems are even more common.[635,636] Virtually every patient with a progressive dementia will have agitation, wandering, sleep difficulties, or other behavioral problems at some point in the course of the disease, and the costs of caring for patients with behavioral symptoms is higher.[637] Therefore, clinicians should proactively discuss behavior and behavioral management with families at the time the dementia is recognized and at subsequent follow-up visits so that the family will be prepared for these developments.

There are several different ways to classify noncognitive behaviors,[638-642] but in the absence of a commonly accepted nosology, the following symptom clusters may be useful in terms of describing symptoms and planning treatments:

- Physical and verbal agitation
- Hallucinations and delusions
- Wandering and pacing
- Symptoms of depression and anxiety
- Sleep disruption
- Eating difficulties.

Some of these categories are purely descriptive, while others use psychiatric terms as "psycho-behavioral metaphors" that acknowledge similarities between behaviors in demented persons and psychiatric syndromes in nondemented persons.[640] These similarities are useful for guiding treatment, but the clinician should be mindful that behavioral symptoms in dementia are manifestations of an older, diseased brain that will usually be far more vulnerable to the side effects of psychiatric medications than the brain of a younger or nondemented patient. In practice, patients will often have combinations of these symptoms or linked symptoms (for example, a patient who paces due to anxiety). Each of these symptom clusters is described in more detail below.

Physical and Verbal Agitation

Agitation describes a variety of disruptive, troublesome behaviors that can be extremely stressful to caregivers and may be presumed to be associated with discomfort among the patients themselves. Types of agitation may include:

- Physical disruption (pushing, hitting, kicking, biting)
- Verbal disruption (screaming, crying) and verbal repetition.

Physical disruption commonly occurs for brief periods of time in the context of care (ie, during bathing or dressing), and this sort of resistiveness to care should be approached differently than spontaneous or unprovoked symptoms.[643] When disruptions consistently occur during a particular activity, these symptoms may respond to modifications of that activity. For example, in the case of a patient who became violent every time his vision was blocked by his t-shirt as it was put on or off over his head by his spouse, simply switching this patient to shirts that buttoned up the front solved the problem of "aggression." Physical disruptions can also occur spontaneously or in response to visual hallucinations, visual misperceptions, visual agnosia (mistaking a family member for a stranger), or delusions.

Persistent yelling or calling out is distressing behavior that is usually associated with more severely impaired patients. If patients cannot express themselves, it is important to perform a physical examination looking for unrecognized sources of pain, particularly bone fractures and dental abscesses, that can easily be overlooked. Repetitive verbalizations, often in the form of a benign question (such as "Where are we going?" or "When are we leaving?"), are not aggressive but can strain the patience of the caregiver.

An uncommon but particularly troubling form of agitation involves persistent sexual comments or hypersexual behavior.

Hallucinations and Delusions

Hallucinations are common symptoms in Alzheimer's disease (AD) and other dementing conditions and are thought to be particularly common and vivid in Lewy body dementias.[664] It can be difficult to differentiate true hallucinations from misperceptions and visual distortions that can occur through the combination of impaired optics and confused cognition. Hallucinations or visual misperceptions often have a paranoid quality, such as when the patient sees vaguely threatening persons in the room or in the yard. If they are primarily misperceptions, better lighting can occasionally reduce the frequency of events.

A delusion is a false, fixed idea. Delusions of danger, abandonment, infidelity, or theft are common as well, causing considerable anxiety and distress. Delusional patients are more prone to agitation, incontinence, wandering, pacing, and disordered sleep.[645] The delusions of dementia often lack consistency and are typically less complex than those in schizophrenia or manic depression.[646]

Wandering and Pacing

Walking actually provides several health benefits for demented persons, preventing the consequences of deconditioning and muscle weakness, reducing the risk of urinary tract infections and pneumonia, and encouraging an experience of independence.[283] But wandering, a general term for inappropriate ambulation, is reported in up to 36% of community-dwelling dementia patients and carries the risk of elopement and falls.[647,648] In cases of wandering, it is always appropriate to ask whether safe outlets for walking can be integrated into the daily life of the patient.

While wandering carries the implication of casual or random walking, pacing is a more driven, nearly constant walking. The precipitants of pacing in an individual patient should always be sought, with particular attention to underlying anxiety, hallucinations, or delusions that could be treated as described in this chapter. Pacing can sometimes be caused by akathisia (restlessness induced by neuroleptics) and may be improved by reducing or stopping those medications. Technological solutions such as wrist activity monitors can measure wandering,[649] while doors with restricted access can limit the dangers of wandering.

Symptoms of Depression and Anxiety

Depressive symptoms often coexist with dementia,[650-652] and these symptoms may be more common in those patients with a family history of mood disorder.[653-654] Early in the course of dementing illnesses, there may be tearfulness, hopelessness, irritability, or somatic complaints (**Table 4.3**). In the later stages, neurovegetative features, such as lack of energy, interest, and appetite, occur and are common to both neurodegenerative dementias and to depression. Anxiety includes feelings of nervousness, worry, and apprehension and may be more common early in dementia when patients are more aware of their deficits. Overstimulation or exposure to unfamiliar situations can sometimes lead to catastrophic reactions with severe anxiety, anger, and aggression.

Estimates vary, but there is general consensus among neuropsychiatric experts that symptoms like these respond to antianxiety or antidepressive treatment in 20% to 40% of demented patients. The full spectrum of major depression or anxiety is not required for demented patients to benefit from medication therapies. Indeed, treatment can reduce the frequency and intensity of symptoms and improve the quality of life for both patient and caregiver.[655] Therefore, we maintain a low threshold for empiric trials of these medications in our demented patients.

Sleep Disruption

Sleep disruption occurs in more than half of community-dwelling AD patients and is one of the most disturbing of the behavioral symptoms associated with AD, creating exhaustion and despair among caregivers.[656,657] In at least one study, sleep disturbances and night wandering were considered among the most intolerable of the behavioral symptoms and thus a major precipitant of institutionalization.[658] Several studies have demonstrated that the average nursing-home resident may never sleep for a full hour, nor be awake for a full hour, throughout the entire 24-hour day.[659,660] Sleep disruption is not only a prominent behavioral problem in patients with AD and other dementias but it may also exacerbate daytime confusion or agitation.

Behaviors characterized by the term "sundowning" are sometimes described along with sleep disruptions, particularly in the nursing home. Sundowning is a widely used term for a clinical phenomenon that is neither medically defined nor biologically understood. In general, sundowning may be characterized by the onset or exacerbation of agitation, restlessness, panic, intensified disorientation, and verbal or physical outbursts in the afternoon or evening. In some studies, disease-related abnormalities of the sleep-wake cycle have been implicated as potential causes of sundowning, although it is clear that patient agitation may contribute to sleep problems as well.[657,661,662]

Eating Difficulties

Eating difficulties can arise at every stage of a dementing illness, and are somewhat more common in patients with more severe dementia, and in those whose caregivers are experiencing the greatest burden.[663] In the early stages, simple weight loss can be caused by an increased caloric need (particularly in patients who are wandering or pacing) or by anorexia from treatment with cholinesterase inhibitors (ChEIs). In moderate-to-severe stages of the dementia, food refusal may signal depression or intercurrent medical illness. Chewing and swallowing difficulties may occur in more advanced stages and can be addressed by providing chopped and pureed food.

Tube feeding is sometimes considered in the latest stages of dementia, although most families and clinicians agree that the quality of life to be sustained at this stage is not desirable. Tube feeding is sometimes advocated to reduce aspiration, but it actually increases the risk of aspiration, deprives patients of the taste of food, may require restraints, and often causes gastrointestinal complications.[664]

Evaluation and Management of Behavioral Symptoms

Whether the patient is living in the community or in an institution, there is no substitute for collecting a careful history of the behavioral symptoms prior to formulating a treatment plan and always before considering medications (**Figure 9.1**). This seemingly simple step is essential for the clinician to even determine whether:

- The caregiver's complaint truly reflects the patient's symptoms or is a cry for help from an overburdened caregiver
- The behavior in question is an isolated occurrence or a frequent event
- Some fundamental feature of the patient's environment or health has changed
- The behavior represents a danger to the patient or to those caring for the patient.

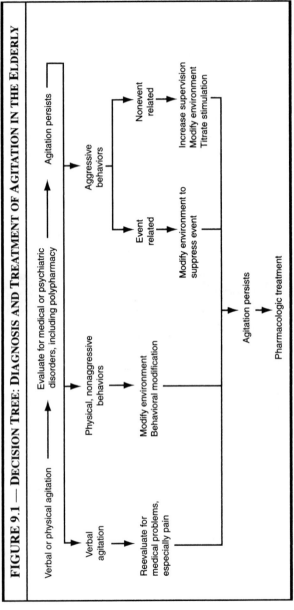

FIGURE 9.1 — DECISION TREE: DIAGNOSIS AND TREATMENT OF AGITATION IN THE ELDERLY

Verbal or physical agitation → Evaluate for medical or psychiatric disorders, including polypharmacy → Agitation persists

Verbal agitation → Reevaluate for medical problems, especially pain

Physical, nonaggressive behaviors → Modify environment / Behavioral modification

Aggressive behaviors

Event related → Modify environment to suppress event

Nonevent related → Increase supervision / Modify environment / Titrate stimulation

Agitation persists → Pharmacologic treatment

160

In moderately and severely impaired patients who are unable to communicate as well, the clinician should specifically consider coincident medical conditions causing increased confusion or pain, particularly occult infections, constipation, hunger, or discomfort from falls.

■ Nonpharmacologic Management Strategies

Nonpharmacological management strategies for agitation and other behaviorial problems should always be considered prior to using medication.[133] In more mildly impaired patients, some behavioral problems represent unrealistic expectations of the patient's abilities and independence on the part of the caregiver and are best addressed by helping the caregiver find a more supervised environment for the patient. For example, a moderately impaired community-dwelling patient with AD who wanders when left alone during the day is usually most appropriately managed by increasing the level of supervision in the home or moving the patient to a more sheltered living arrangement. In other situations, simple behavioral interventions may be remarkably effective—as with the restriction of evening fluids and regular toileting to avoid nighttime bathroom confusion or scheduling supervised mall trips for a patient who likes to wander. In community dwelling patients with AD, an exercise program combined with caregiver education improved physical health and depression symptoms in the AD patients.[665] In nursing homes and special care units, environmental modifications can have significant effects on moderating behaviors.[666] General suggestions for nonpharmacologic management of troublesome behaviors are shown in **Table 9.1** and are reviewed elsewhere.[667,668]

TABLE 9.1 — NONPHARMACOLOGIC INTERVENTIONS FOR BEHAVIORAL SYMPTOMS IN DEMENTIA

- Increase supervision
- Minimize visual deficits with good lighting and prescription glasses
- Minimize auditory deficits by reducing background noise, speaking clearly, and obtaining hearing aids if necessary
- Minimize fatigue by scheduling rest periods
- Use signage and directions for patients who can still read
- Use reassurance, distraction, and redirection for emotional outbursts
- Increase or decrease visual, auditory, or social stimulation
- Provide formal or informal activity programs
- Reduce or avoid naps if nighttime sleep is a problem
- Schedule regular toileting to reduce incontinence or nighttime agitation associated with bathroom needs
- Modify the environment with:
  - Bedside toilets
  - Night lights
  - Door locks or alarms
  - Identification bracelets or tags
  - Safe places to wander
  - Current photographs of patient and loved ones for reference
- Teach caregivers how to manage behaviors and support daily activities

■ Pharmacologic Management Strategies

If environmental changes and nonpharmacologic interventions are unsuccessful, medications can be used to address behavior abnormalities. Even when medications are used, the principles of nonpharmacologic management should continue to be applied and the need for medications should be regularly reevaluated.

Current practices for medication management of behavioral symptoms in dementia rely upon clinical experience, an evolving understanding of the neurochemistry of dementia, and certain parallels between these symptoms and psychiatric syndromes in nondemented persons. Several different approaches have been described,[640,668-673] and there are no clear-cut procedures for choosing medications. However, **Table 9.2** summarizes pharmacological treatment of behavioral disturbances. No matter which medications are chosen, general principles of pharmacologic treatment include the following:

- Use low doses of all psychoactive medications and increase slowly
- Consider non-neuroleptics first
- Avoid the use of multiple medications when possible
- Reevaluate the need for and the dosage of medication frequently.

Typical Neuroleptics

Typical neuroleptics include haloperidol, thioridazine, trifluoperazine, and chlorpromazine. These have the advantage of being familiar to most clinicians and are inexpensive, but may sometimes induce orthostatic hypotension or parkinsonian side effects, including problems with gait and posture that can lead to falls. Haloperidol has minimal anticholinergic side effects and produces only mild sedation. Many clinicians have

TABLE 9.2 — PSYCHOTROPIC AGENTS USEFUL FOR THE TREATMENT OF NEUROPSYCHIATRIC SYMPTOMS AND BEHAVIORAL DISTURBANCES IN PATIENTS WITH ALZHEIMER'S DISEASE

Type/Generic Drug (Trade) Name	Initial Daily Dose	Final Daily Dose (Range)	Targeted Symptoms
Atypical antipsychotic			Psychosis and agitation
Risperidone (Risperdal)	0.5 mg/d	1.0 mg (0.75-1.5 mg/d)	
Olanzapine (Zyprexa)	2.5 mg/d	5.0 mg (5-10 mg/d)	
Quetiapine (Seroquel)	25 mg/d	200 mg (50-150 mg bid)	
Ziprasidone (Geodon)	20 mg/d	40 mg (20-80 mg bid)	
Aripiprazole (Abilify)	10 mg/d	10 mg (10-30 mg/d)	
Neuroleptic			Psychosis and agitation
Haloperidol (Haloperidol, others)	0.25 mg/d	2 mg (1-3 mg/d)	
Mood stabilizer			Agitation
Divalproex sodium (Depakote)	125 mg bid	500 mg (250-500 mg bid)	
Carbamazepine (Tegretol, others)	200 mg bid	400 mg (200-500 mg bid)	

Selective serotonin reuptake inhibitor			Depression, anxiety, psychosis, and agitation
Citalopram (Celexa)	10 mg/d	20 mg (20-40 mg/d)	
Escitalopram (Lexapro)	5 mg/d	10 mg (10-20 mg/d)	
Paroxetine (Paxil)	10 mg/d	20 (10-40 mg/d)	
Sertraline (Zoloft)	25 mg/d	75 mg (75-100 mg/d)	
Fluoxetine (Prozac, others)	5 mg/d	10 mg (10-40 mg/d)	
Tricyclic antidepressant			Depression
Nortriptyline (Pamelor, others)	10 mg/d	50 mg (25-100 mg/d)	
Desipramine (Norpramin, others)	10 mg/d	100 mg (50-200 mg/d)	
Serotonin- and noradrenergic-reuptake inhibitor			Depression and anxiety
Venlafaxine (Effexor)	25 mg bid	200 mg (100-150 mg bid)	
Noradrenergic and specific serotonergic antidepressant			Depression
Mirtazapine (Remeron, others)	7.5 mg/d	15 mg (15-30 mg/d)	

Cummings JL. *N Engl J Med*. 2004;351:64.

9

traditionally used low-dose haloperidol at a dosage of 0.5 mg to 1 mg once or twice a day to reduce the frequency or intensity of agitation in conjunction with hallucinations or delusions. If this regimen is used, carefully reexamine the patient weekly for a few weeks, then every few months to make sure parkinsonian side effects do not occur. While at least one well-designed study that showed no benefit for haloperidol or trazodone over placebo,[674] another showed benefit for haloperidol and tiapride vs placebo,[675] and in general, these medications are felt to have efficacy.[676]

Atypical Neuroleptics

The newer, atypical neuroleptics include risperidone, olanzapine, clozapine, and quetiapine, with others in development. The advantage of these medications is that they are far less likely to be associated with parkinsonian side effects than the typical neuroleptics.[677] In rare cases, these medications can also induce parkinsonian features, but they have become the first-line pharmacologic treatments for some forms of agitation because side effects are relatively low. We have the most experience with risperidone (starting at 0.5 mg to 1 mg every other day and slowly increasing to 2 mg bid if necessary) and olanzapine (starting at 5 mg qd and increasing to 10 mg qd, if necessary); we have avoided using clozapine because of the risk of agranulocytosis that requires monitoring of white blood cell counts. The primary side effect of the atypical neuroleptics is sedation, and this is useful in treating agitation that occurs at night. An excellent review of this literature and more detailed information on dosing and side effects is available elsewhere.[673]

Antidepressants

The use of selective serotonin reuptake inhibitors is typically safe, even in older persons, and can be quite effective for elevating or stabilizing depressed or labile mood, or for blunting symptoms of agitation and anxiety. It is often helpful to initiate antidepressant treatment in the face of fragmentary symptoms of depression even if the full syndrome is not present.[678] In every case, start these at the lowest starting dosage recommended and gradually increase to a typical, but low, antidepressant dosage. For example, we will often start a patient on sertraline 25 mg daily, increasing to 50 mg daily, and if necessary, increasing further to 100 mg daily.

The antidepressant trazodone is frequently used for the treatment of agitation, particularly if sleep problems are involved. We typically begin with a low dose of 50 mg at bedtime and increase slowly up to 100 mg bid. We add the morning dose only to impact daytime agitation, and if the problem is largely restricted to nighttime, increase only the evening dose.

Tricyclic antidepressants are rarely used because of the added confusion that can occur with the anticholinergic properties of these medications. However, occasionally a low dose of nortriptyline or doxepin at bedtime is useful to aid sleep in a demented patient without causing additional confusion.

9

Anxiolytics

While some clinicians use benzodiazepines (ie, short-acting lorazepam), particularly in acute situations, we typically avoid them as they can lower inhibitions and add to confusion. However, buspirone is an anxiolytic with less sedative properties that is sometimes used for the long-term management of agitation or anxiety, usually starting at 5 mg bid and increasing to 10 mg to 25 mg bid.

Anticonvulsants

In recent years, trials have demonstrated that anticonvulsants, particularly carbamazepine and valproic acid, have efficacy for stabilizing mood disorders and other psychiatric conditions. There is evidence that these medications may be effective in reducing agitation and aggression among demented patients as well,[679] although randomized controlled trials have not always shown significance.[680-683]

Other Medications

As described in Chapter 8, *Current and Emerging Therapies*, the ChEIs appear to provide significant behavioral improvement.[684-689] β-Blockers, particularly propranolol and pindolol, have also been used to treat physical aggressiveness and motor restlessness in demented patients, but efficacy is less well documented and the risk of adverse effects in terms of heart disease makes this a less favorable choice. Other medications that have been reported to help include opioids,[690] for agitation. Melatonin has been proposed for the treatment of sleep disruption but has not been shown to be helpful.[691]

10 Family Education and Support

The family members of a patient with Alzheimer's disease (AD) and other progressive dementias lose their loved one in a prolonged process that robs the patient of precious shared memories, the ability to appreciate care, and eventually, autonomy and dignity. It often seems that family members suffer even more than patients, but the involvement of family members goes far beyond simply becoming additional victims of the disease. Family members form the interface between the patient and the world, filtering the patient's experiences and in later stages, structuring every moment of the patient's day. As the disease progresses, it is the family members who eventually decide on everything from medication schedules to nursing-home placement.

Thus the clinician who works to educate and support family members is not just showing empathy for the feelings of persons related to the patient but dramatically improving the quality of life for that patient. Providing a diagnosis, then waiting for the family to call with problems, is no more appropriate with AD than it would be with diabetes or heart disease. *Specific planning for family education and support is a fundamental and essential component in the management of patients with dementia.* While this need not be done by the same clinician who has diagnosed or is medically managing the dementing illness, planning should include:

- Holding formal educational sessions with family members at each stage of the disease (not

just handing out pamphlets or referral to the Alzheimer's Association)
- Monitoring the mental and physical health of the family members caring for the patient.

Caregiving "Career" and Caregiver Stress

In most families, a spouse or adult child assumes the role of the "primary caregiver," an unanticipated and demanding job with "no salary, benefits, sick days or vacations."[692] Stages of caregiving include the encounter stage, when the diagnosis is received and the family struggles to adjust; the enduring stage, in which there is frequently fatigue, isolation, and depression; and the exit stage, as family members face both grief and relief at the prospect of long-term care and death.[692] As this chapter focuses largely upon the difficulties of caregiving, it should also be kept in mind that this new role can, in some cases, also provide a sad but rewarding outlet for expressing love and for bringing families closer together.

At any stage of a dementing disease, the caregivers can become isolated and exhausted, and experience high rates of anxiety, depression, physical deterioration, and even death.[693,694] All caregivers are vulnerable, but those who are younger, less well educated, with lower incomes, and must care for behaviorally disturbed loved ones are particularly more likely to become depressed.[695] When caregivers themselves are uninformed or overwhelmed, patients experience more behavioral problems and require nursing-home placement earlier.[696] Ethnic minorities may be reluctant to use formal support services and rely instead upon extended networks of family and friends.[697] Financially and educationally disadvantaged families will have fewer resources and options for support. Supporting the family members, especially the primary caregiver, requires a full interdisciplinary approach that should be coordinated by the primary-care clinician and, at different stages of the disease, will usually include:

- Educating the family about what to expect at each stage in the illness
- Coordinating medical information with other clinical specialists
- Encouraging caregivers to take care of their own emotional and health needs
- Providing informal counseling and sometimes psychotherapy referral to the caregiver
- Alerting families to financial, legal, and insurance issues
- Referring the family to the Alzheimer's Association for education and support groups
- Providing recommendations for formal or informal home-based care services (providing assistance with housekeeping, meals, and transportation).

The use of education and support groups deserves special mention because there is evidence that these services reduce psychiatric and physical morbidity in caregivers.[698] In fact, in a study in which families were randomized to receive counseling and participate in active weekly support groups, those who received the intervention were able to maintain the affected family member longer in the home.[447]

Communicating With Patients and Caregivers

As discussed in Chapter 3, *Evaluation of the Older Patient With Cognitive Problems*, Chapter 8, *Current and Emerging Therapies*, and Chapter 9, *Man-*

agement of Agitation and Behavioral Symptoms, clinicians should solicit clinical information from family members and include them in all treatment decisions. While it may seem awkward at first, creating an opportunity to speak to the family *without the patient in the room* facilitates this, both at the initial evaluation and during subsequent visits, and we routinely do this at all visits. In a practice setting, the patient can be examined by one clinician (ie, a nurse who is administering a standardized cognitive measure like the Mini-Mental State Examination [MMSE]) while another speaks to family members. Despite the anticipated concerns of family members when separated from the demented person, patients themselves rarely object to waiting for a few moments alone. The front office staff can be trained to monitor the patient in the waiting area at such times in case the patient wanders or becomes upset while the clinician is meeting with the family. At every appointment, meetings with multiple family members (not just the primary caregiver) should be sought so that the clinician can gain insight into the caregiving dynamics of the particular family. Family members should always be informed and reminded of the definitive or suspected diagnoses ("Last time we told you that we strongly suspected the diagnosis of Alzheimer's disease, and your husband's continued decline now confirms that diagnosis."). Imprecise diagnostic labels, such as dementia, or outmoded terms, such as senility, should be avoided.

Simply confirming the diagnosis, even when it has been previously suspected, is such an emotional shock to family members that they may not remember much of what is discussed. We routinely send them home with written comments and recommendations that they can review and share with other family members who did not come to the appointment. Family members are often concerned that the clinician not upset the patient by naming the specific diagnosis, particularly AD, in their presence. We find that the patient's memory disorder makes this problem moot in all but the earliest cases of the disease. However, families feel so strongly about this that unless specifically asked by the patient, we do not mention the specific disorder of AD to him or her. After discussion with the family, we typically bring the patient back into the room and explain to the patient that he or she has a memory problem, then outline the steps we are taking to treat that problem.

In subsequent appointments, the clinician can provide an overview of the disease and of the medical options and support services that will be available. When treatments are recommended for symptomatic improvement of cognitive symptoms (Chapter 8, *Current and Emerging Therapies*) or for the management of behavioral problems (Chapter 9, *Management of Agitation and Behavioral Symptoms*), follow-up appointments to monitor those issues are excellent opportunities to assess how the family is coping and provide further assistance. The management of the patient with AD may begin with a highly functioning, even fully employed patient, and continue until death, spanning as long as 20 years! The best education and management is often that which is one step ahead of the disease process, so it is essential to schedule regular appointments at least every 6 months, even when the demented patient has few active medical issues. By keeping in such steady contact with patients and families, clinicians can help families at critical junctures as they try to maintain a safe environment, confront the patient's driving and financial privileges, and respond to the escalating necessity for supervised care—often culminating in the agonizing decision to place the patient in a nursing home.

Safety Issues

Almost any behavior can pose a risk to an individual with dementia. Examples of potentially dangerous events include leaving the house alone, wandering, dressing inappropriately for the cold, becoming lost, using a toaster or a stove improperly, and eating spoiled food. Even when the demented person can perform routine activities without difficulty, confusion may hamper his or her ability to respond appropriately to an unexpected or dangerous situation, such as an electrical problem in the home or a simple fall. Persons with cognitive impairment can easily become the victims of financial scams or be taken advantage of by unscrupulous family members. Safety in the home can be increased by emphasizing home safeguards and caregiver competence. As the dementia worsens, the simplest, but sometimes most difficult, intervention is to gradually increase direct supervision. However, since many demented patients live independently in the early stages of their disease, a few key safeguards should always be considered:

- Reducing fire hazards by putting timers on stoves and ovens
- Reducing medication errors by counting pills into pillboxes
- Reducing falls by adding handrails and changing loose rugs
- Reducing and stopping driving by the patient.

Driving

Restricting the driving privileges of patients with dementia deserves special mention because it is such an emotionally charged issue in many families. Regardless of what patients and their families may claim, as a group, persons with even mild dementia drive more poorly and have a greater risk of accidents than persons without dementia.[699-701] Yet, in the very earliest stages of dementia when memory problems are the only detectable deficits, many patients appear to drive safely on familiar streets, and the symbolic impact of reducing a patient's independence by preventing the patient from driving can be distressing and divisive within a family.

The decision to restrict or forbid driving on the basis of cognitive impairment is best made jointly by the family and the clinician since patients routinely resist surrendering this privilege, even when they are obviously too impaired to drive safely. The discussion should include:

- Patient's capacity and competence
- Patient's driving history
- Current driving patterns
- Transportation needs
- Potential alternative means for transportation.

There are no rules to help clinicians judge when to restrict patient driving and the neuropsychologic heterogeneity of a disease like AD means that mildly impaired patients with visuospatial problems may be more dangerous on the road than patients with severe, but more straightforward, amnestic problems. However, our clinical experience and some published literature[701] suggest that problems are under-reported by caregivers,[702] and that driving should be seriously examined and probably curtailed in patients whose MMSE scores decline below 25. In questionable cases, a standardized driving evaluation from a rehabilitation center, driving school, or local department of motor vehicles may help determine some aspects of driver competence. But in progressive dementias, such a snapshot does not accurately reflect what the patient will be like several months later, or even the next day, since there is such day-to-day fluctuation in concentration of impaired patients.

When the impairments are very mild, the clinician can wean the patient from driving by encouraging the family to find other alternatives and gradually begin using them well before driving must be terminated. When driving privileges must be restricted suddenly, a carefully worded statement implying that the loss of privilege will be temporary ("I'm afraid you will need to stop driving while we work on ways to help your memory problem.") is not entirely honest but often softens the blow. The clinician can also relieve pressure within the family by accepting the blame for the restriction, and since the amnestic patient will quickly forget the conversation, the responsibility of the clinician can be reinforced if he or she writes the words "Do not drive" on a prescription pad and sends this "prescription" home with the patient as a reminder. These recommendations should also be applied to patients who operate heavy machinery or who possess guns in the home.[703]

Financial and Legal Issues

If a progressive dementia is recognized in the early stages, family members should be encouraged to seek the patient's guidance in making long-term financial and legal decisions while the patient can still comprehend and participate. A good elder law attorney can be particularly helpful. Such planning may include:

- Establishing durable power of attorney for financial matters
- Including a family member's name on bank accounts
- Financing of home-health or institutional care
- Completing or updating of patient's last will and testament

- Planning a living will and durable power of attorney for health care or health-care proxy, with advanced directives such as restrictions on resuscitation measures.

As the patient with progressive dementia loses cognitive function, he or she may be unable to accurately make important financial and legal decisions. Assessing capacity has been proposed as a means of evaluating ability to make decisions about finances,[704] participation in research,[705] or voting.[706] Financial issues are usually the most problematic, and while the caregiver can become either a limited or full legal guardian of the patient, a simpler and less costly step is to establish durable power of attorney while the patient still has sufficient cognitive capability to agree to and sign such an agreement. This gives the caregiver legal power to make financial and medical decisions on behalf of the patient.

The differences between a *last will and testament* and a *living will* are frequently misunderstood. A last will and testament is a legal document that expresses how property and wealth are divided after death. A living will is a document that is used to state the patient's preferences about certain medical procedures that could be used to postpone or prolong death. A living will is usually designed to indicate a patient's preferences to die naturally without extensive measures, such as tube feeding or cardiopulmonary resuscitation.

Respite Care

Respite care provides essential physical and emotional support for caregivers, serving the dual purpose of decreasing the burden of care and allowing caregivers to continue to work or fulfill other responsibilities.[698] The respite may occur at any stage of the disease, may be ongoing or intermittent, may last for hours to weeks, and may be provided informally or programmatically by:

- Family members or friends
- Home-health aides or visiting nurses
- Day-care programs
- Brief nursing-home stays.

Day-care programs are particularly valuable in the mild-to-moderate stages of the disease, but caregivers are often so exhausted and stressed that they need considerable encouragement to explore any of these options. These programs can usually be found through local social workers, senior-service and community organizations, local churches, and the local chapter of the Alzheimer's Association.

Residential-Care Facilities

Persons with AD and other progressive dementing illnesses can be cared for at home or in residential sites that provide a continuum of care (**Figure 10.1**). In the early stages of dementia, living in community settings (where some help and oversight are provided, but there is usually no on-site staff) or assisted-living facilities (where on-site assistance is provided) may be a good alternative. Both of these options require private pay from residents or their families. Facilities in the same category may have very different staffing plans. Some will have no formal caregivers, while others will have elaborate interdisciplinary teams of case managers along with medical and activity staffing. Social workers, geriatric case managers, and local chapters of the Alzheimer's Association are good referral sources to share with families who are trying to evaluate the merits of different residential facilities, but there is no substitute for the families visiting the facility themselves

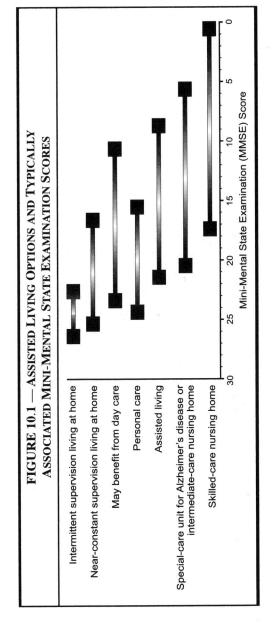

FIGURE 10.1 — ASSISTED LIVING OPTIONS AND TYPICALLY ASSOCIATED MINI-MENTAL STATE EXAMINATION SCORES

Intermittent supervision living at home

Near-constant supervision living at home

May benefit from day care

Personal care

Assisted living

Special-care unit for Alzheimer's disease or intermediate-care nursing home

Skilled-care nursing home

Mini-Mental State Examination (MMSE) Score

179

and discussing the philosophy and resources with the staff.

As the patient with progressive dementia becomes more dependent, the burden of caregiving grows, and in the moderate-to-severe stages, patients will no longer be able to be supported in assisted-living environments. Most families will not have the physical or financial means to maintain the patient in the home. Caregivers desperately hope to avoid nursing-home placement and sometimes avoid discussion or planning for it until exhaustion or illness overwhelms them and a crisis erupts. Clinicians can help families considerably by introducing the possibilities for long-term care as a contingency well before it is required. This way, family members can select and apply for a suitable facility, plan for payment, and make emotional adjustments to this step.

The immediate precipitants to residential placement are typically one or more of the following:[707]
- Disruptive and uncooperative behaviors
- Bladder and bowel incontinence
- Sleep disturbances
- Failure of patient to recognize the caregiver
- Withdrawal of an assisting, paid caregiver
- Caregiver illness or "burnout."

Most traditional nursing homes are modeled after hospitals, focusing on medical illness and medical management. However, in recent years, a wide variety of residential facilities for demented persons have been built and marketed, including special facilities that specifically cater to patients with AD. Since Medicare does not cover the costs of long-term facilities, families must pay for these out of pocket (or through previously purchased long-term care insurance). In the case of traditional nursing-home care, the patient must qualify on the basis of financial need for enrollment in a Medicaid nursing home.

Starting in the 1970s, thousands of nursing homes established special-care units (SCUs) in which demented residents are segregated from the mainstream residents.[708,709] The principal motivation for the establishment of these SCUs has been to better meet the needs of cognitively impaired residents. However, in some cases, the segregation of demented and disruptive residents is done to provide more aesthetic conditions for the nondemented residents, while in others, this label appears to be little more than a marketing strategy.[710] Ideally, residential units that specialize in the care of dementia patients should provide comfortable, less clinical environments, focused activities and staffing patterns to promote the functional abilities of demented residents, environmental designs that allow residents to wander safely, and opportunities for the active involvement of family members. Some facilities encourage the residence of the nondemented spouse, and others include several levels of supervised care so that a patient who becomes too demented for one level can move to a more intensive level without leaving the facility altogether.

In summary, without uniform guidelines, funding structures, or even nomenclature, every family must individually negotiate the challenges of finding a suitable residential facility and the traumas of moving the patient out of the home, often in the face of bitter opposition and accusations by the patient. To assist families with this task, clinicians should obtain and distribute lists and summaries of local facilities and contacts and urge families to visit and join the waiting list of appropriate facilities well before the decision is necessary.

10

Hospice Care

For AD patients who are terminally ill (generally life expectancy of 6 months or less), hospice care may be an option.[707] Such care must be prescribed by a clinician and may follow either home or institutional care. Many medical centers and hospitals now offer hospice care, either institutionally or at home. Home-based care is usually provided by:

- A nurse, who provides medical attention
- A social worker, who provides support and counseling to patient and caregiver
- A home-health aid, who assists with bathing and grooming.

Humane assistance from these services can provide great comfort to families in the last few weeks or months of a patient's life. Whether or not hospice care is utilized, the death of the patient with AD is often a relief to the caregiver, and symptoms of depression in caregivers can actually improve after the patient's demise.[711] Clinicians can help families of dying AD patients through the terminal phases of the disease by offering awareness and support through the intellectual and emotional conflicts that occur.[712]

11 Resources for Clinicians and Families

General Information on Alzheimer's Disease

Alzheimer's Association (National Headquarters)
225 N. Michigan Avenue, 17th Floor
Chicago, IL 60601
Phone: 800-272-3900 or 312-335-8700
Website: www.alz.org

Alzheimer's Disease Education & Referral Center
PO Box 8250
Silver Spring, MD 20907-8250
Phone: 800-438-4380
Website: www.alzheimers.org

Alzheimer's Disease International
45/46 Lower Marsh
London SE1 7RG, United Kingdom
Phone: 44 20 7620 3011
Website: www.alz.co.uk

Alzheimer's Foundation of America
322 8th Avenue, 6th Floor
New York, NY 10001
Phone: 866-AFA-8484
Websites: www.alzfdn.org; www.careprofessionals.org

Information on Research in Alzheimer's Disease

Alzheimer Research Forum
Website: www.alzforum.org

Boston University Alzheimer's Disease Center
Phone: 888-458-BUAD (2823)
Websites: www.bualzresearch.com

National Library of Medicine, NIH Clinical Trials
Website: www.clinicaltrials.gov

Information on Health and Aging-Related Services

Administration on Aging
Washington, DC 20201
Phone: 800-677-1116 or 202-619-0724
ElderCare Locator 800-677-1116
Websites: www.aoa.dhhs.gov; www.eldercare.gov

American Association of Homes and
  Services for the Aging
2519 Connecticut Ave, NW
Washington, DC 20008
Phone: 202-783-2242
Website: www.aahsa.org

American Bar Association
Commission on Law and Aging
740 Fifteenth Street, NW
Washington, DC 20005-1022
Phone: 202-662-8690
Website: www.abanet.org/aging

American Health Care Association
1201 L Street NW
Washington, DC 20005
Phone: 800-321-0343 or 202-842-4444
Website: www.ahca.org

American Health Assistance Foundation
22512 Gateway Center Dr.
Clarksburg, MD 20871
Phone: 800-437-2423 or 301-948-3244
Website: www.ahaf.org

American Society on Aging
833 Market Street, Suite 511
San Francisco, CA 94103-1824
Phone: 415-974-9600
Website: www.asaging.org

Centers for Medicare & Medical Services
Phone: 800-MEDICARE
Website: www.medicare.gov

Elderweb
1305 Chadwick Drive
Normal, IL 61761
Phone: 309-451-3319
Website: www.elderweb.com

Family Caregiver Alliance
690 Market Street, Suite 600
San Francisco, CA 94104
Phone: 415-434-3388
Website: www.caregiver.org

National Academy of Elder Law Attorneys
1604 North Country Club Road
Tucson, Arizona 85716
Phone: 520-881-4005
Website: www.naela.org

National Association of Area Agencies on Aging
927 15th Street, NW, 6th floor
Washington, DC 20005
Phone: 202-296-8130
Website: www.n4a.org

National Council on Aging
300 D Street, SW
Suite 801
Washington, DC 20024
Phone: 800-424-9046 or 202-479-1200
Website: www.ncoa.org

11

National Hospice and Palliative Care Organization
1700 Diagonal Road, Suite 625
Alexandria, VA 22314
Phone: 703-837-1500
Website: www.nhpco.org

National Institute on Aging
Building 31, Room 5C27
31 Center Drive, MSC 2292
Bethesda, MD 20892
Phone: 800-222-2225 or 301-496-1752
Website: www.nia.nih.gov; www.nihseniorhealth.gov

National Library of Medicine, NIH
Website: www.medlineplus.gov

Social Security Administration
Phone: 1-800-772-1213
General Website: www.ssa.gov
Website for Seniors: www.seniors.gov

Books — Patient Activities

Abrignani C, Messinger B. *Alzheimer's Disease: Activities That Work.* La Grange, Tex: M & H Publishing Company; 1991.

ADEAR Center. *Alzheimer's Disease: Unraveling the Mystery.* Silver Springs, Md: ADEAR Center; 2002.

Alzheimer's Association. *Activity Programming for Persons With Dementia: A Sourcebook.* Chicago, Ill: Alzheimer's Association; 1995.

Dowling JR. *Keeping Busy: A Handbook of Activities for Persons With Dementia.* Baltimore, Md: Johns Hopkins University Press; 1995.

Books — Behavioral Management

Hinman-Smith E, Gwyther LP. *Coping With Challenging Behaviors: Education Strategies for Work With Alzheimer's Families.* Durham, NC: Duke University Medical Center; 1990.

Journeyworks Publishing. Brochures with tips for caregivers such as *Dealing With Wandering, Sleeping Through the Night, Making Mealtime Easier, Caring for the Caregiver,* and *Making Communication Easier for a Person with Memory Loss and Confusion.* Santa Cruz, Calif.

Robinson A, Spencer B, White L. *Understanding Difficult Behaviors: Some Practical Suggestions for Coping With Alzheimer's Disease and Related Illness.* Ypsilanti, Mich: Eastern Michigan University and Alzheimer's Care and Training Center; 1989.

Books — Caregiving

ADEAR Center. *Caregiver Guide: Tips for Caregivers of People with Alzheimer's Disease.* Silver Springs, Md: ADEAR Center; 2001.

ADEAR Center. *Home Safety for People with Alzheimer's Disease.* Silver Springs, Md: ADEAR Center; 2002.

American Association for Geriatric Psychiatry. *Caring for the Alzheimer's Disease Patient: How You Can Provide the Best Care and Maintain Your Own Well-Being.* Bethesda, Md: American Association for Geriatric Psychiatry; 2003.

Coon DW, Gallagher-Thompson D, Thompson LW. *Innovative Interventions to Reduce Dementia Caregiver Distress: A Clinical Guide.* New York, NY: Springer Publishing Company, Inc; 2003.

Coste JK. *Learning to Speak Alzheimer's: A Ground-Breaking Approach for Everyone Dealing with the Disease.* Boston, Mass: Houghton Mifflin; 2003.

Karr KL. *Taking Time for Me: How Caregivers Can Effectively Deal With Stress.* Buffalo, NY: Prometheus Books; 1992.

Gruetzner H. *A Caregiver's Guide and Sourcebook.* New York, NY: John Wiley and Sons Inc; 1991.

11

Journeyworks. *Caring for a Person With Memory Loss and Confusion: An Easy Guide for Caregivers.* Santa Cruz, Calif: Journeyworks Publishing; 2002.

Mace NL, Rabins PV. *The 36-Hour Day: A Family Guide to Caring for Persons With Alzheimer's Disease, Related Dementing Illnesses and Memory Loss in Later Life.* 3rd ed. Baltimore, Md: The Johns Hopkins University Press; 1999.

Medina J. *What You Need to Know About Alzheimer's.* New York, NY: New Harbinger Publications; 1999.

Mittleman MS, Epstein C. *Alzheimer's Health Care Handbook: How to Get the Best Medical Care for Your Relative With Alzheimer's Disease, In and Out of the Hospital.* New York, NY: Marlowe and Company; 2002.

Mittleman MS. *Counseling the Alzheimer's Caregiver.* Chicago, Ill: American Medical Association Press; 2003.

Rader J, Tornquist EM. *Individualized Dementia Care: Creative Compassionate Approach.* New York, NY: Springer Publishing Company; 1995.

Richter RW, Richter BZ. *Alzheimer's Disease: A Physicians Guide to Practical Management.* Totowa, NJ: Humana Press; 2004.

Roberts DJ. *Taking Care of Caregivers: For Families and Others Who Care for People With Alzheimer's Disease and Other Forms of Dementia.* Palo Alta, Calif: Bull Publishing; 1991.

Warner ML. *Complete Guide to Alzheimer's-Proofing Your Home.* West Lafayette, Ind: Purdue University Press; 1998.

Books — Communication

Hodgson H. *Alzheimer's: Finding the Words: A Communication Guide for Those Who Care.* Minneapolis, Minn: Chronimed Publishing; 1995.

Lubinski R. *Dementia and Communication.* Philadelphia, Pa: Decker; 1991.

Books — Early and Late Stages

ADEAR Center. *Reflections on Memories Lost: Stories of Early Alzheimer's Disease With Expert Commentary on Symptoms, Diagnosis and Treatment from Dr. John C. Morris.* Silver Springs, Md: ADEAR Center; 2002.

Kuhn D. *Alzheimer's Early Stages: First Steps for Family, Friends & Caregivers. 2nd ed.* Alamedia, Calif; 2003.

Volicer L, Hurley A. *Hospice Care for Patients With Advanced Progressive Dementia.* New York, NY: Springer Publishing Company; 1998.

Books — Written by Persons With Alzheimer's Disease

Davis R. *My Journey Into Alzheimer's Disease.* Wheaton, Ill: Tyndale House Publishing; 1999.

Rose L. *Show Me the Way to Go Home.* Forest Knolls, Calif: Elder Books; 1996.

Snyder L. *Speaking our Minds: Personal Reflections from Individuals with Alzheimers.* New York, NY: WH Freeman Publishers; 2000.

11

Materials Written for the Person
With Alzheimer's Disease

Alzheimer's Association. *If You Have Alzheimer's Disease: What You Should Know, What You Should Do.* Chicago, Ill: Alzheimer's Association; 1998.

Alzheimer's Association Canada. *Just for You: For People Diagnosed With Alzheimer's Disease.* Toronto, ON: Alzheimer Canada; 1997.

Davies HD, Jensen MP. *Alzheimer's: The Answers You Need.* Forest Knolls, Calif: Elder Books; 1998.

CD-ROM for Caregivers

Burns T, Hepburn K, Maddox M, Smith SL. *Alzheimer's Caregiving Strategies.* To purchase:
HealthCare Interactive
PO Box 19646
Minneapolis, MN 55419
1-888-824-3020

Local Resources

Alzheimer's Association Chapters

Tel: _____

Tel: _____

Tel: _____

Social Services

Tel: _____

Tel: _____

Geriatric Case Managers

Tel: _____

Tel: _____

Tel: _____

Geriatric/Behavioral Neurologists

Tel: _____

Tel: _____

Tel: _____

Geriatric/Psychiatrists

Tel: _____

Tel: _____

Tel: _____

11

12 References

1. Bureau of Census. 1996.
2. Green RC. Alzheimer's disease and other dementing disorders. In: Joynt R, ed. *Clinical Neurology*. Philadelphia, Pa: Lippencott-Raven; 1995:1-84.
3. Cummings JL, Benson DF. *Dementia: A Clinical Approach*. Boston, Mass: Butterworth-Heinemann; 1992.
4. Powell AL. Senile dementia of extreme aging: a common disorder of centenarians. *Dementia*. 1994;5:106-109.
5. Louhija J, Miettinen HE, Kontula K, Tikkanen MJ, Miettinen TA, Tilvis RS. Aging and genetic variation of plasma apolipoproteins. Relative loss of the apolipoprotein E4 phenotype in centenarians. *Arterioscler Thromb*. 1994;14:1084-1089.
6. Forette B. Centenarians: health and frailty. In: Robine J-M, Vaupel JW, Jeune B, Allard M, eds. *Longevity: To the Limits and Beyond*. Berlin: Springer-Verlag; 1997:105-112.
7. Petersen RC, Smith GE, Waring SC, Ivnik RJ, Tangalos EG, Kokmen E. Mild cognitive impairment: clinical characterization and outcome [published correction appears in *Arch Neurol*. 1999;56:760]. *Arch Neurol*. 1999;56:303-308.
8. American Psychiatric Association. *Diagnostic and Statistical Manual of Mental Disorders, Revised Fourth Edition*. Washington, DC: American Psychiatric Association; 1995.
9. Katzman R, Kawas C. Epidemiology of dementia and Alzheimer disease. In: Terry RD, Katzman R, Bick KL, eds. *Alzheimer Disease*. New York, NY: Raven Press, Ltd; 1994:105-122.
10. Farrer LA. Genetics and the dementia patient. *The Neurologist*. 1997;3:13-30.
11. Jorm AF, Korten AE, Henderson AS. The prevalence of dementia: a quantitative integration of the literature. *Acta Psychiatr Scand*. 1987;76:465-479.
12. Rocca WA, Bonaiuto S, Lippi A, et al. Prevalence of clinically diagnosed Alzheimer's disease and other dementing disorders: a door-to-door survey in Appignano, Macerata Province, Italy. *Neurology*. 1990;40:626-631.
13. Zhang MY, Katzman R, Salmon D, et al. The prevalence of dementia and Alzheimer's disease in Shanghai, China: impact of age, gender, and education. *Ann Neurol*. 1990;27:428-437.
14. Fukunishi I, Hayabara T, Hosokawa K. Epidemiological surveys of senile dementia in Japan. *Int J Soc Psychiatry*. 1991;37:51-56.
15. Fratiglioni L, Grut M, Forsell Y, et al. Prevalence of Alzheimer's disease and other dementias in an elderly urban population: relationship with age, sex, and education. *Neurology*. 1991;41:1886-1892.
16. Ueda K, Kawano H, Hasuo Y, Fujishima M. Prevalence and etiology of dementia in a Japanese community. *Stroke*. 1992;23:798-803.
17. Aronson MK, Ooi WL, Geva DL, Masur D, Blau A, Frishman W. Dementia. Age-dependant incidence, prevalence, and mortality in the old old. *Arch Intern Med*. 1991;151:989-992.

12

18. Shibayama H, Kasahara Y, Kobayashi H. Prevalence of dementia in a Japanese elderly population. *Acta Psychiatr Scand.* 1986;74:144-151.

19. O'Connor DW, Pollitt PA, Hyde JB, et al. The prevalence of dementia as measured by the Cambridge Mental Disorders of the Elderly Examination. *Acta Psychiatr Scand.* 1989;79:190-198.

20. Evans DA, Funkenstein HH, Albert MS, et al. Prevalence of Alzheimer's disease in a community population of older persons. Higher than previously reported. *JAMA.* 1989;262:2551-2556.

21. Heeren TJ, Lagaay AM, Hijmans W, Rooymans HG. Prevalence of dementia in the 'oldest old' of a Dutch community. *J Am Geriatr Soc.* 1991;39:755-759.

22. Aronson MK, Ooi WL, Geva DL, Masur D, Blau A, Frishman W. Dementia. Age-dependent incidence, prevalence, and mortality in the old old. *Arch Intern Med.* 1991;151:989-992.

23. Skoog I, Nilsson L, Palmertz B, Andreasson LA, Svanborg A. A population-based study of dementia in 85-year-olds. *N Engl J Med.* 1993;328:153-158.

24. Ebly EM, Parhad IM, Hogan DB, Fung TS. Prevalence and types of dementia in the very old: results from the Canadian Study of Health and Aging. *Neurology.* 1994;44:1593-1600.

25. Wernicke TF, Reischies FM. Prevalence of dementia in old age: clinical diagnoses in subjects aged 95 years and older. *Neurology.* 1994;44:250-253.

26. Johansson B, Zarit SH. Prevalence and incidence of dementia in the oldest old: a longitudinal study of a population-based sample of 84-90 year-olds in Sweden. *Int J Geriatr Psychiatry.* 1995;10:359-366.

27. Ritchie K, Ledésert B, Touchon J. The Eugéria study of cognitive aging: who are the "normal" elderly. *Int J Geriatr Psychiatry.* 1993;8:969-977.

28. Ritchie K, Kildea D. Is senile dementia "age-related" or "ageing-related"? Evidence from meta-analysis of dementia prevalence in the oldest old. *Lancet.* 1995;346:931-934.

29. Perls TT. The oldest old. *Sci Am.* 1995;272:70-75.

30. Breitner JC, Wyse BW, Anthony JC, et al. APOE-ε4 count predicts age when prevalence of AD increases, then declines: the Cache County Study. *Neurology.* 1999;53:321-331.

31. Hebert LE, Scherr PA, Bienias JL, Bennett DA, Evans DA. Alzheimer disease in the US population: prevalence estimates using the 2000 census. *Arch Neurol.* 2003;60:1119-1122.

32. Wimo A, Winblad B, Aguero-Torres H, von Strauss E. The magnitude of dementia occurrence in the world. *Alzheimer Dis Assoc Disord.* 2003;17:63-67.

33. Bachman DL, Wolf PA, Linn RT, et al. Incidence of dementia and probable Alzheimer's disease in a general population: the Framingham Study. *Neurology.* 1993;43:515-519.

34. Hebert LE, Scherr PA, Beckett LA, et al. Age-specific incidence of Alzheimer's disease in a community population. *JAMA.* 1995;273:1354-1359.

35. Aevarsson O, Skoog I. A population-based study on the incidence of dementia disorders between 85 and 88 years of age. *J Am Geriatr Soc.* 1996;44:1455-1460.

36. Lopez-Pousa S, Vilalta-Franch J, Llinas-Regla J, Garre-Olmo J, Roman GC. Incidence of dementia in a rural community in Spain: the Girona cohort study. *Neuroepidemiology.* 2004;23:170-177.

37. Hendrie HC, Ogunniyi A, Hall KS, et al. Incidence of dementia and Alzheimer disease in 2 communities: Yoruba residing in Ibadan, Nigeria, and African Americans residing in Indianapolis, Indiana. *JAMA*. 2001;285:739-747.

38. Bowirrat A, Treves TA, Friedland RP, Korczyn AD. Prevalence of Alzheimer's type dementia in an elderly Arab population. *Eur J Neurol*. 2001;8:119-123.

39. Miech RA, Breitner JC, Zandi PP, Khachaturian AS, Anthony JC, Mayer L. Incidence of AD may decline in the early 90s for men, later for women: The Cache County study. *Neurology*. 2002;58:209-218.

40. Prince M, Acosta D, Chiu H, Scazufca M, Varghese M; 10/66 Dementia Research Group. Dementia diagnosis in developing countries: a cross-cultural validation study. *Lancet*. 2003;361:909-917.

41. Jorm AF. Cross-national comparisons of the occurrence of Alzheimer's and vascular dementias. *Eur Arch Psychiatry Clin Neurosci*. 1991;240:218-222.

42. Livingston G, Sax K, Willison J, Blizard B, Mann A. The Gospel Oak Study stage II: the diagnosis of dementia in the community. *Psychol Med*. 1990;20:881-891.

43. Cummings JL, Benson DF. Dementia: definition, prevalence, classification and approach to diagnosis. *Dementia: A Clinical Approach*. Boston, Mass: Butterworth-Heinemann; 1992:6.

44. Small GW, Rabins PV, Barry PP, et al. Diagnosis and treatment of Alzheimer's disease and related disorders. Consensus statement of the American Association for Geriatric Psychiatry, the Alzheimer's Association, and the American Geriatrics Society. *JAMA*. 1997;278:1363-1371.

45. American Psychiatric Association. Practice guideline for the treatment of patients with Alzheimer's disease and other dementias of late life. *Am J Psychiatry*. 1997;154(suppl 5):1-39.

46. Strub RL, Black FW. *The Mental Status Examination in Neurology*. Philadelphia, Pa: FA Davis; 1993.

47. Bachman DL, Green RC. Speech and language disorders. In: Hurst JW, ed. *Medicine for the Practicing Physician*. 3rd ed. Boston, Mass: Butterworth-Heinemann; 1992:1684-1687.

48. Folstein MF, Folstein SE, McHugh PR. "Mini-mental state." A practical method for grading the cognitive state of patients for the clinician. *J Psychiatr Res*. 1975;12:189-198.

49. Folstein M, Anthony JC, Parhad I, Duffy B, Gruenberg EM. The meaning of cognitive impairment in the elderly. *J Am Geriatr Soc*. 1985;33:228-235.

50. Anthony JC, LeResche L, Niaz U, von Korff MR, Folstein MF. Limits of the 'Mini-Mental State' as a screening test for dementia and delirium among hospital patients. *Psychol Med*. 1982;12:397-408.

51. Pfeffer RI, Kurosaki TT, Harrah C, et al. A survey diagnostic tool for senile dementia. *Am J Epidemiol*. 1981;114:515-527.

52. Nelson A, Fogel BS, Faust D. Bedside cognitive screening instruments. A critical assessment. *J Nerv Ment Dis*. 1986;174:73-83.

53. Schwamm LH, Van Dyke C, Kiernan RJ, Murrin EL, Mueller J. The Neurobehavioral Cognitive Status Examination: comparison with the Cognitive Capacity Screening Examination and the Mini-Mental State Examination in a neurosurgical population. *Ann Intern Med*. 1987; 107:486-491.

12

54. Faustman WO, Moses JA Jr, Csernasnsky JG. Limitations of the Mini-Mental State Examination in predicting neuropsychological functioning in a psychiatric sample. *Acta Psychiatr Scand.* 1990;81: 126-131.

55. Applegate WB, Blass JP, Williams TF. Instruments for the functional assessment of older patients. *N Engl J Med.* 1990;322:1207-1214.

56. Murrell SA, Himmelfarb S, Wright K. Prevalence of depression and its correlates in older adults. *Am J Epidemiol.* 1983;117:173-185.

57. Yesavage JA, Brink TL, Rose TL, et al. Development and validation of a geriatric depression screening scale: a preliminary report. *J Psychiatr Res.* 1983;17:37-49.

58. Yesavage JA. Geriatric depression scale. *Psychopharmacol Bull.* 1988;24:709-711.

59. Weintraub S. Neuropsychological assessment of mental state. In: Mesulam M-M, ed. *Principles of Cognitive and Behavioral Neurology.* 2nd ed. New York, NY: Oxford University Press; 2000:121-173.

60. Albert MS, Moss MB. *Geriatric Neuropsychology.* New York, NY: Guilford Press; 1988.

61. Heilman KM, Valenstein E. *Clinical Neuropsychology.* 3rd ed. New York, NY: Oxford University Press; 1993.

62. Albert MS. Age-related changes in cognitive function. In: Albert ML, Knoefel JE, eds. *Clinical Neurology of Aging.* 2nd ed. New York, NY: Oxford University Press; 1994:314-346.

63. de Leon MJ, Golomb J, George AE, et al. The radiologic prediction of Alzheimer disease: the atrophic hippocampal formation. *Am J Neuroradiol.* 1993;14:897-906.

64. Killiany RJ, Moss MB, Albert MS, Sandor T, Tieman J, Jolesz F. Temporal lobe regions on magnetic resonance imaging identify patients with early Alzheimer's disease. *Arch Neurol.* 1993;50:949-954.

65. Jack CR Jr, Petersen RC, Xu Y, et al. Rates of hippocampal atrophy correlate with change in clinical status in aging and AD. *Neurology.* 2000;55:484-489.

66. Killiany RJ, Hyman BT, Gomez-Isla T, et al. MRI measures of entorhinal cortex vs hippocampus in preclinical AD. *Neurology.* 2002;58:1188-1196.

67. Braffman BH, Zimmerman RA, Trojanowski JQ, Gonatas NK, Hickey WF, Schlaepfer WW. Brain MR: pathologic correlation with gross and histopathology. 2. Hyperintense white-matter foci in the elderly. *Am J Roentgenol.* 1988;151:559-566.

68. Janota I, Mirsen TR, Hachinski VC, Lee DH, Merskey H. Neuropathologic correlates of leuko-araiosis [published correction appears in *Arch Neurol.* 1990;47:281]. *Arch Neurol.* 1989;46:1124-1128.

69. Moody DM, Brown WR, Challa VR, Anderson RL. Periventricular venous collagenosis: association with leukoaraiosis. *Radiology.* 1995;194:469-476.

70. Burger LJ, Rowan AJ, Goldensohn ES. Creutzfeldt-Jakob disease. An electroencephalographic study. *Arch Neurol.* 1972;26:428-433.

71. Traub RD, Pedley TA. Virus-induced electrotonic coupling: hypothesis on the mechanism of periodic EEG discharges in Creutzfeldt-Jakob disease. *Ann Neurol.* 1981;10:405-410.

72. Reiman EM, Caselli RJ, Yun LS, et al. Preclinical evidence of Alzheimer's disease in persons homozygous for the epsilon 4 allele for apolipoprotein E. *N Engl J Med.* 1996;334:752-758.

73. Jagust W, Thisted R, Devous MD Sr, et al. SPECT perfusion imaging in the diagnosis of Alzheimer's disease: a clinical-pathologic study. *Neurology.* 2001;56:950-956.

74. Osimani A, Ichise M, Chung DG, Pogue JM, Freedman M. SPECT for differential diagnosis of dementia and correlation of rCBF with cognitive impairment. *Can J Neurol Sci.* 1994;21:104-111.

75. Foster NL. PET imaging. In: Terry RD, Katzman R, Bick KL, eds. *Alzheimer Disease.* New York, NY: Raven Press, Ltd; 1994:87-103.

76. Weiner MF, Wighton-Benn WH, Risser R, et al. Xenon-133 SPECT-determined regional cerebral blood flow in Alzheimer's disease: what is typical? *J Neuropsychiatry Clin Neurosci.* 1993;5:415-418.

77. Alzheimer's disease: a statistical approach using positron emission to-mographic data. *J Cereb Blood Flow Metab.* 1993;13:438-447.

78. Pietrini P, Azari NP, Grady CL, et al. Pattern of cerebral metabolic interactions in a subject with isolated amnesia at risk for Alzheimer's disease: a longitudinal evaluation. *Dementia.* 1993;4:94-101.

79. Bookheimer SY, Strojwas MH, Cohen MS, et al. Patterns of brain activation in people at risk for Alzheimer's disease. *N Engl J Med.* 2000;343:450-456.

80. Reiman EM, Chen K, Alexander GE, et al. Functional brain abnormalities in young adults at genetic risk for late-onset Alzheimer's dementia. *Proc Natl Acad Sci USA.* 2004;101:284-289.

81. Klunk WE, Engler H, Nordberg A, et al. Imaging brain amyloid in Alzheimer's disease with Pittsburgh Compound-B. *Ann Neurol.* 2004;55:306-319.

82. Small GW, Agdeppa ED, Kepe V, Satyamurthy N, Huang SC, Barrio JR. In vivo brain imaging of tangle burden in humans. *J Mol Neurosci.* 2002;19:323-327.

83. Herholz K. PET studies in dementia. *Ann Nucl Med.* 2003;17:79-89.

84. Nordberg A. PET imaging of amyloid in Alzheimer's disease. *Lancet Neurol.* 2004;3:519-527.

85. Small GW, Mazziotta JC, Collins MT, et al. Apolipoprotein E type 4 allele and cerebral glucose metabolism in relatives at risk for familial Alzheimer disease. *JAMA.* 1995;273:942-947.

86. Wolfe N, Reed BR, Eberling JL, Jagust WJ. Temporal lobe perfusion on single photon emission computed tomography predicts the rate of cognitive decline in Alzheimer's disease. *Arch Neurol.* 1995;52:257-262.

87. Woodard JL, Grafton ST, Votaw JR, Green RC, Dobraski ME, Hoffman JM. Compensatory recruitment of neural resources during overt rehearsal of word lists in Alzheimer's disease. *Neuropsychology.* 1998;12:491-504.

88. Green RC, Goldstein FC, Mirra SS, Alazraki NP, Baxt JL, Bakay RA. Slowly progressive apraxia in Alzheimer's disease. *J Neurol Neurosurg Psychiatry.* 1995;59:312-315.

89. Miller BL, Cummings JL, Villanueva-Meyer J, et al. Frontal lobe de-generation: clinical, neuropsychological, and SPECT characteristics. *Neurology.* 1991;41:1374-1382.

90. Tyrrell PJ, Sawle GV, Ibanez V, et al. Clinical and positron emission tomographic studies in the 'extrapyramidal syndrome' of dementia of the Alzheimer type. *Arch Neurol.* 1990;47:1318-1323.

91. Waltregny A, Maula AA, Brucher JM. Contribution of stereotactic brain biopsies to the diagnosis in several cases of dementia. *Acta Neurol Belg.* 1989;89:161-167.

12

92. Hulette CM, Earl NL, Crain BJ. Evaluation of cerebral biopsies for the diagnosis of dementia. *Arch Neurol.* 1992;49:28-31.

93. Clarfield AM. The decreasing prevalence of reversible dementias: an updated meta-analysis. *Arch Intern Med.* 2003;163:2219-2229.

94. Grossman I, Kaufman AS, Mednitsky S, Scharff L, Dennis B. Neurocognitive abilities for a clinically depressed sample versus a matched control group of normal individuals. *Psychiatry Res.* 1994;51:231-244.

95. Brown RG, Scott LC, Bench CJ, Dolan RJ. Cognitive function in depression: its relationship to the presence and severity of intellectual decline. *Psychol Med.* 1994;24:829-847.

96. Stoudemire A, Hill C, Gulley LR, Morris R. Neuropsychological and biomedical assessment of depression-dementia syndromes. *J Neuropsychiatry Clin Neurosci.* 1989;1:347-361.

97. Folstein MR, Rabins PV. Replacing pseudodementia. *Neuropsychiatry Neuropsychol Behav Neurol.* 1991;4:36-40.

98. Tatemichi TK. How acute brain failure becomes chronic: a view of the mechanisms of dementia related to stroke. *Neurology.* 1990;40:1652-1659.

99. Brust JC. Vascular dementia is overdiagnosed. *Arch Neurol.* 1988;45:799-801.

100. O'Brien JT, Erkinjuntti T, Reisberg B, et al. Vascular cognitive impairment. *Lancet Neurol.* 2003;2:89-98.

101. Gorelick PB, Brody J, Cohen D, et al. Risk factors for dementia associated with multiple cerebral infarcts. A case-control analysis in predominantly African-American hospital-based patients. *Arch Neurol.* 1993;50:714-720.

102. Tatemichi TK, Desmond DW, Paik M, et al. Clinical determinants of dementia related to stroke. *Ann Neurol.* 1993;33:568-575.

103. Hachinski VC, Lassen NA, Marshall J. Multi-infarct dementia. A cause of mental deterioration in the elderly. *Lancet.* 1974;2:207-210.

104. Hachinski VC, Iliff LD, Zilhka E, et al. Cerebral blood flow in dementia. *Arch Neurol.* 1975;32:632-637.

105. Rosen WG, Terry RD, Fuld PA, Katzman R, Peck A. Pathologic verification of ischemic score in differentiation of dementias. *Ann Neurol.* 1980;7:486-488.

106. Moroney JT, Bagiella E, Desmond DW, et al. Meta-analysis of the Hachinski Ischemic Score in pathologically verified dementias. *Neurology.* 1997;49:1096-1105.

107. Roman GC, Erkinjuntti T, Wallin A, Pantoni L, Chui HC. Subcortical ischaemic vascular dementia. *Lancet Neurol.* 2002;1:426-436.

108. Mirsen T, Hachinski V. The epidemiology and classification of vascular and multi-infarct dementia. In: Meyer JS, Lechner H, Marshall J, Toole JF, eds. *Vascular and Multi-Infarct Dementia.* Mount Kisco, NY: Futura; 1988:61-76.

109. Roman GC, Tatemichi TK, Erkinjuntti T, et al. Vascular dementia: diagnostic criteria for research studies. Report of the NINDS-AIREN International Workshop. *Neurology.* 1993;43:250-260.

110. Chui HC, Victoroff JI, Margolin D, Jagust W, Shankle R, Katzman R. Criteria for the diagnosis of ischemic vascular dementia proposed by the State of California Alzheimer's Disease Diagnostic and Treatment Centers. *Neurology.* 1992;42:473-480.

111. World Health Organization. *The ICD-10 Classification of Mental and Behavioural Disorders: Clinical Descriptions and Diagnostic Guidelines.* Geneva, Switzerland: WHO; 1992:50-51.

112. Gold G, Giannakopoulous P, Montes-Paixao C, et al. Sensitivity and specificity of newly proposed clinical criteria for possible vascular dementia. *Neurology.* 1997;49:690-694.

113. Snowdon DA, Greiner LH, Mortimer JA, Riley KP, Greiner PA, Markesbery WR. Brain infarction and the clinical expression of Alzheimer disease. The Nun Study. *JAMA.* 1997;277:813-817.

114. Orrison WW, Glastonburg CM. Adult white matter disease. In: Orrison WW, ed. *Neuroimaging.* Philadelphia: WB Saunders; 2000:800-828.

115. Gunning-Dixon FM, Raz R. The cognitive correlates of white matter abnormalities in normal aging: a quantitative review. *Neuropsychology.* 2000;14:224-232.

116. Smith CD, Snowdon DA, Wang H, Markesbery WR. White matter volumes and periventricular white matter hyperintensities in aging and dementia. *Neurology.* 2000;54:838-842.

117. de Groot JC, de Leeuw FE, Oudkerk M, Hofman A, Jolles J, Breteler MM. Cerebral white matter lesions and depressive symptoms in elderly adults. *Arch Gen Psychiatry.* 2000;57:1071-1076.

118. Benson RR, Guttmann CR, Wei X, et al. Older people with impaired mobility have specific loci of periventricular abnormality on MRI. *Neurology.* 2002;58:48-55.

119. Bigler ED, Lowry CM, Kerr B, et al. Role of white matter lesions, cerebral atrophy, and APOE on cognition in older persons with and without dementia: the Cache County, Utah, study of memory and aging. *Neuropsychology.* 2003;17:339-352.

120. Weller RO, Nicoll JA. Cerebral amyloid angiopathy: pathogenesis and effects on the ageing and Alzheimer brain. *Neurol Res.* 2003;25:611-616.

121. Love S, Nicoll JA, Hughes A, Wilcock GK. APOE and cerebral amyloid angiopathy in the elderly. *Neuroreport.* 2003;14:1535-1536.

122. Natte R, Maat-Schieman ML, Haan J, Bornebroek M, Roos RA, van Duinen SG. Dementia in hereditary cerebral hemorrhage with amyloidosis-Dutch type is associated with cerebral amyloid angiopathy but is independent of plaques and neurofibrillary tangles. *Ann Neurol.* 2001;50:765-772.

123. O'Donnell HC, Rosand J, Knudsen KA, et al. Apolipoprotein E genotype and the risk of recurrent lobar intracerebral hemorrhage. *N Engl J Med.* 2000;342:240-245.

124. Nicoll JA, McCarron MO. APOE gene polymorphism as a risk factor for cerebral amyloid angiopathy-related hemorrhage. *Amyloid.* 2001;8(suppl 1):51-55.

125. Eng JA, Frosch MP, Choi K, Rebeck GW, Greenberg SM. Clinical manifestations of cerebral amyloid angiopathy-related inflammation. *Ann Neurol.* 2004;55:250-256.

126. Dichgans M, Mayer M, Uttner I, et al. The phenotypic spectrum of CADASIL: clinical findings in 102 cases. *Ann Neurol.* 1998;44:731-739.

127. Auer DP, Putz B, Gossl C, Elbel G, Gasser T, Dichgans M. Differential lesion patterns in CADASIL and sporadic subcortical arteriosclerotic encephalopathy: MR imaging study with statistical parametric group comparison. *Radiology.* 2001;218:443-451.

12

128. Joutel A, Andreux F, Gaulis S, et al. The ectodomain of the Notch3 receptor accumulates within the cerebrovasculature of CADASIL patients. *J Clin Invest.* 2000;105:597-605.

129. Chabriat H, Bousser MG. CADASIL. Cerebral autosomal dominant arteriopathy with subcortical infarcts and leukoencephalopathy. *Adv Neurol.* 2003;92:147-150.

130. Forette F, Seux ML, Stassen JA, et al. Prevention of dementia in randomised double-blind placebo-controlled Systolic Hypertension in Europe (Syst-Eur) trial. *Lancet.* 1998;352:1347-1351.

131. Erkinjuntti T, Kurz A, Gauthier S, Bullock R, Lilienfeld S, Damaraju CV. Efficacy of galantamine in probable vascular dementia and Alzheimer's disease combined with cerebrovascular disease: A randomised trial. *Lancet.* 2002;359:1283-1290.

132. Black S, Roman GC, Geldmacher DS, et al. Efficacy and tolerability of donepezil in vascular dementia: positive results of a 24-week, multicenter, international, randomized, placebo-controlled clinical trial. *Stroke.* 2003;34:2323-2330.

133. Doody RS, Stevens JC, Beck C, et al. Practice parameter: management of dementia (an evidence-based review). Report of the Quality Standards Subcommittee of the American Academy of Neurology. *Neurology.* 2001;56:1154-1166.

134. Winblad B, Palmer K, Kivipelto M, et al. Mild cognitive impairment—beyond controversies, towards a consensus: report of the International Working Group on Mild Cognitive Impairment. *J Intern Med.* 2004;256:240-246.

135. Mobius HJ, Stoffler A. New approaches to clinical trials in vascular dementia: memantine in small vessel disease. *Cerebrovasc Dis.* 2002;13(suppl 2):S61-S66.

136. Wilcock G, Mobius H, Stoffler A; MMM 500 group. A double-blind, placebo-controlled multicentre study of memantine in mild to moderate vascular dementia (MMM500). *Int Clin Psychopharmacol.* 2002;17:297-305.

137. Mayeux R, Stern Y, Rosenstein R, et al. An estimate of the prevalence of dementia in idiopathic Parkinson's disease. *Arch Neurol.* 1988;45:260-262.

138. Snow B, Wiens M, Hertzman C, Calne D. A community survey of Parkinson's disease. *CMAJ.* 1989;141:418-422.

139. Aarsland D, Andersen K, Larsen JP, Lolk A, Kragh-Sorensen P. Prevalence and characteristics of dementia in Parkinson disease: an 8-year prospective study. *Arch Neurol.* 2003;60:387-392.

140. Noe E, Marder K, Bell KL, Jacobs DM, Manly JJ, Stern Y. Comparison of dementia with Lewy bodies to Alzheimer's disease and Parkinson's disease with dementia. *Mov Disord.* 2004;19:60-67.

141. Colosimo C, Hughes AJ, Kilford L, Lees AJ. Lewy body cortical involvement may not always predict dementia in Parkinson's disease. *J Neurol Neurosurg Psychiatry.* 2003;74:852-856.

142. McKeith IG, Mosimann UP. Dementia with Lewy bodies and Parkinson's disease. *Parkinsonism Relat Disord.* 2004;10 (suppl 1):S15-S18.

143. McKeith IG, Galasko D, Kosaka K, et al. Consensus guidelines for the clinical and pathologic diagnosis of dementia with Lewy bodies (DLB): report of the consortium on DLB international workshop. *Neurology.* 1996;47:1113-1124.

144. Perry R, McKeith I, Perry E. *Dementia With Lewy Bodies*. Cambridge, UK: Cambridge University Press; 1996.

145. Lippa CF, McKeith I. Dementia with Lewy bodies: improving diagnostic criteria. *Neurology*. 2003;60:1571-1572.

146. McKeith IG, Fairbairn AF, Perry RH, Thompson P. The clinical diagnosis and misdiagnosis of senile dementia of Lewy body type (SDLT). *Br J Psychiatry*. 1994;165:324-332

147. Hohl U, Tiraboschi P, Hansen LA, Thal LJ, Corey-Bloom J. Diagnostic accuracy of dementia with Lewy bodies. *Arch Neurol*. 2000;57:347-351.

148. Merdes AR, Hansen LA, Jeste DV, et al. Influence of Alzheimer pathology on clinical diagnostic accuracy in dementia with Lewy bodies. *Neurology*. 2003;60:1586-1590.

149. Wild R, Pettit T, Burns A. Cholinesterase inhibitors for dementia with Lewy bodies. Cochrane Database of Systemic Reviews 3. 2003: CD003672.

150. Kaufer DI. Pharmacologic treatment expectations in the management of dementia with Lewy bodies. *Dement Geriatr Cogn Disord*. 2004;17(suppl 1):32-39.

151. Mann DM, South PW, Snowden JS, Neary D. Dementia of frontal lobe type: neuropathology and immunohistochemistry. *J Neurol Neurosurg Psychiatry*. 1993;56:605-614.

152. Miller BL, Darby A, Benson DF, Cummings JL, Miller MH. Aggressive, socially disruptive and antisocial behavior in frontotemporal dementia. *Br J Psychiatry*. 1997;170:150-154.

153. Levy ML, Miller BL, Cummings JL, Fairbanks LA, Craig A. Alzheimer's disease and frontotemporal dementia. Behavioral distinctions. *Arch Neurol*. 1996;53:687-690.

154. The Lund and Manchester Groups. Clinical and neuropathological criteria for frontotemporal dementia. *J Neurol Neurosurg Psychiatry*. 1994;57:416-418.

155. Brun A, Passant U. Frontal lobe degeneration of non-Alzheimer type. Structural characteristics, diagnostic criteria and relation to other frontotemporal dementias. *Acta Neurol Scand Suppl*. 1996;168(suppl): 28-30.

156. Neary D, Snowden JS, Gustafson L, et al. Frontotemporal lobar degeneration: a consensus on clinical diagnostic criteria. *Neurology*. 1998;51:1546-1554.

157. Varma AR, Snowden JS, Lloyd JJ, Talbot PR, Mann DM, Neary D. Evaluation of the NINCDS-ADRDA criteria in the differentiation of Alzheimer's disease and frontotemporal dementia. *J Neurol Neurosurg Psychiatry*. 1999;66:184-188.

158. Snowden JS, Neary D, Mann DMA. *Fronto-temporal Lobar Degeneration*. New York, NY: Churchill-Livingstone; 1996.

159. Ratnavalli E, Brayne C, Dawson K, Hodges JR. The prevalence of frontotemporal dementia. *Neurology*. 2002;58:1615-1621.

160. Rosen HJ, Hartikainen KM, Jagust W, et al. Utility of clinical criteria in differentiating frontotemporal lobar degeneration (FTLD) from AD. *Neurology*. 2002;58:1608-1615.

161. Chow TW, Miller BL, Hayashi VN, Geschwind DH. Inheritance of frontotemporal dementia. *Arch Neurol*. 1999;56:817-822.

162. Hutton M, Lendon CL, Rizzu P, et al. Association of missense and 5'-splice-site mutations in tau with the inherited dementia FTDP-17. *Nature*. 1998;393:702-705.

12

163. Kertesz A. Pick's complex and FTDP-17. *Mov Disord.* 2003;18(suppl 6):S57-S62.

164. Morris HR, Khan MN, Janssen JC, et al. The genetic and pathological classification of familial frontotemporal dementia. *Arch Neurol.* 2001;58:1813-1816.

165. Steinbart EJ, Smith CO, Poorkaj P, Bird TD. Impact of DNA testing for early-onset familial Alzheimer disease and frontotemporal dementia. *Arch Neurol.* 2001;58:1828-1831.

166. Prusiner SB. Human prion diseases and neurodegeneration. *Curr Top Microbiol Immunol.* 1996;207:1-17.

167. Brown P, Cathala F, Castaigne P, Gajdusek DC. Creutzfeldt-Jakob disease: clinical analysis of a consecutive series of 230 neuropathologically verified cases. *Ann Neurol.* 1986;20:597-602.

168. Cambier DM, Kantarci K, Worrell GA, Westmoreland BF, Aksamit AJ. Lateralized and focal clinical, EEG, and FLAIR MRI abnormalities in Creutzfeldt-Jakob disease. *Clin Neurophysiol.* 2003;114:1724-1728.

169. Lemstra AW, van Meegen MT, Vreyling JP, et al. 14-3-3 testing in diagnosing Creutzfeldt-Jakob disease: a prospective study in 112 patients. *Neurology.* 2000;55:514-516.

170. Zerr I, Pocchiari M, Collins S, et al. Analysis of EEG and CSF 14-3-3 proteins as aids to the diagnosis of Creutzfeldt-Jakob disease. *Neurology.* 2000;55:811-815.

171. Huang N, Marie SK, Livramento JA, Chammas R, Nitrini R. 14-3-3 protein in the CSF of patients with rapidly progressive dementia. *Neurology.* 2003;61:354-357.

172. EUROCJD Group. Genetic epidemiology of Creutzfeldt-Jakob disease in Europe. *Rev Neurol* (Paris). 2001;157:633-637.

173. Goldman JS, Miller BL, Safar J, et al. When sporadic disease is not sporadic: the potential for genetic etiology. *Arch Neurol.* 2004;61:213-216.

174. Jason GW, Pajurkova EM, Suchowersky O, et al. Presymptomatic neuropsychological impairment in Huntington's disease. *Arch Neurol.* 1988;45:769-773.

175. Spencer MD, Knight RS, Will RG. First hundred cases of variant Creutzfeldt-Jakob disease: retrospective case note review of early psychiatric and neurological features. *BMJ.* 2002;324:1479-1482.

176. Irani DN. The classic and variant forms of Creutzfeldt-Jakob disease. *Semin Clin Neuropsychiatry.* 2003;8:71-79.

177. Ho AK, Sahakian BJ, Brown RG, et al; NEST-HD Consortium. Profile of cognitive progression in early Huntington's disease. *Neurology.* 2003;61:1702-1706.

178. The Huntington's Disease Collaborative Research Group. A novel gene containing a trinucleotide repeat that is expanded and unstable on Huntington's disease chromosomes. *Cell.* 1993;72:971-983.

179. Duyao M, Ambrose C, Myers R, et al. Trinucleotide repeat length instability and age of onset in Huntington's disease. *Nat Genet.* 1993;4:387-392.

180. Went L, Broholm J, Cassiman J, Craufurd D. Guidelines for the molecular genetics predictive test in Huntington's disease. *Neurology.* 1994;44:1533-1536.

181. Bonelli RM, Wenning GK, Kapfhammer HP. Huntington's disease: present treatments and future therapeutic modalities. *Int Clin Psychopharmacol.* 2004;19:51-62.

182. McArthur JC, Hoover DR, Bacellar H, et al. Dementia in AIDS patients: incidence and risk factors. Multicenter AIDS Cohort Study. *Neurology.* 1993;43:2245-2252.

183. Ho DD, Bredesen DE, Vinters HV, Daar ES. The acquired immunodeficiency syndrome (AIDS) dementia complex. *Ann Intern Med.* 1989;111:400-410.

184. Navia BA, Cho ES, Petito CK, Price RW. The AIDS dementia complex: II. Neuropathology. *Ann Neurol.* 1986;19:525-535.

185. Wesselingh SL, Thompson KA. Immunopathogenesis of HIV-associated dementia. *Curr Opin Neurol.* 2001;14:375-379.

186. Nath A. Human immunodeficiency virus (HIV) proteins in neuropathogenesis of HIV dementia. *J Infect Dis.* 2002;186(suppl 2):S193-S198.

187. Price RW, Brew BJ. The AIDS dementia complex. *J Infect Dis.* 1988;158:1079-1083.

188. Koralnik IJ. New insights into progressive multifocal leukoencephalopathy. *Curr Opin Neurol.* 2004;17:365-370.

189. van Duijn CM, Clayton D, Chandra V, et al. Familial aggregation of Alzheimer's disease and related disorders: a collaborative reanalysis of case-control studies. EURODEM Risk Factors Research Group. *Int J Epidemiol.* 1991;20(suppl 2):S13-S20.

190. Lautenschlager NT, Cupples LA, Rao VS, et al. Risk of dementia among relatives of Alzheimer's disease patients in the MIRAGE study: what is in store for the oldest old? *Neurology.* 1996;46:641-650.

191. Green RC, Cupples LA, Go R, et al. Risk of dementia among white and African American relatives of patients with Alzheimer disease. *JAMA.* 2002;287:329-336.

192. Cupples LA, Farrer LA, Sadovnick AD, Relkin N, Whitehouse P, Green RC. Estimating risk curves for first-degree relatives of patients with Alzheimer's disease: the REVEAL study. *Genet Med.* 2004;6:192-196.

193. Farrer LA, Cupples LA, Haines JL, et al. Effects of age, sex and ethnicity on the association between apolipoprotein E genotype and Alzheimer disease. A meta-analysis. APOE and Alzheimer Disease Meta Analysis Consortium. *JAMA.* 1997;278:1349-1356.

194. Rao VS, Cupples A, van Duijn CM, et al. Evidence for major gene inheritance of Alzheimer disease in families of patients with and without apolipoprotein E ε4. *Am J Hum Genet.* 1996;59:664-675.

195. Katzman R. Education and the prevalence of dementia and Alzheimer's disease. *Neurology.* 1993;43:13-20.

196. Guo Z, Cupples LA, Kurz A, et al. Head injury and the risk of Alzheimer disease in the MIRAGE Study. *Neurology.* 2000;54:1316-1323.

197. Roberts GW, Allsop D, Bruton C. The occult aftermath of boxing. *Neuropathol Appl Neurobiol.* 1989;15:273-274.

198. Teasdale GM, Nicoll JA, Murray G, Fiddes M. Association of apolipoprotein E polymorphism with outcome after head injury. *Lancet.* 1997;350:1069-1071.

199. Friedman G, Froom P, Sazbon L, et al. Apolipoprotein E-epsilon 4 genotype predicts a poor outcome in survivors of traumatic brain injury. *Neurology.* 1999;52:244-248.

200. Honig LS, Tang MX, Albert S, et al. Stroke and the risk of Alzheimer disease. *Arch Neurol.* 2003;60:1707-1712.

201. Lee PN. Smoking and Alzheimer's disease: a review of the epidemiological evidence. *Neuroepidemiology.* 1994;13:131-144.

12

202. Tyas SL, White LR, Petrovitch H, et al. Mid-life smoking and late-life dementia: the Honolulu-Asia Aging Study. *Neurobiol Aging*. 2003;24:589-596.

203. Aronson MK, Ooi WL, Morgenstern H, et al. Women, myocardial infarction, and dementia in the very old. *Neurology*. 1990;40:1102-1106.

204. Sparks DL, Hunsaker JC 3d, Scheff SW, Kryscio RF, Henson JL, Markesbery WR. Cortical senile plaques in coronary artery disease, aging and Alzheimer's disease. *Neurobiol Aging*. 1990;11:601-607.

205. Ravona-Springer R, Davidson M, Noy S. The role of cardiovascular risk factors in Alzheimer's disease. *CNS Spectr*. 2003;8:824-833.

206. Qiu C, Winblad B, Viitanen M, Fratiglioni L. Pulse pressure and risk of Alzheimer disease in persons aged 75 years and older: a community-based, longitudinal study. *Stroke*. 2003;34:594-599.

207. Qiu C, Winblad B, Fastbom J, Fratiglioni L. Combined effects of APOE genotype, blood pressure, and antihypertensive drug use on incident AD. *Neurology*. 2003;61:655-660.

208. Ott A, Stolk RP, van Harskamp F, Pols HA, Hofman A, Breteler MM. Diabetes mellitus and the risk of dementia: The Rotterdam Study. *Neurology*. 1999;53:1937-1942.

209. Luchsinger JA, Tang MX, Stern Y, Shea S, Mayeux R. Diabetes mellitus and risk of Alzheimer's disease and dementia with stroke in a multiethnic cohort. *Am J Epidemiol*. 2001;154:635-641.

210. Arvanitakis Z, Wilson RS, Bienias JL, Evans DA, Bennett DA. Diabetes mellitus and risk of Alzheimer disease and decline in cognitive function. *Arch Neurol*. 2004;61:661-666.

211. Tan ZS, Seshadri S, Beiser A, et al. Plasma total cholesterol level as a risk factor for Alzheimer disease: the Framingham Study. *Arch Intern Med*. 2003;163:1053-1057.

212. Reitz C, Tang MX, Luchsinger J, Mayeux R. Relation of plasma lipids to Alzheimer disease and vascular dementia. *Arch Neurol*. 2004;61:705-714.

213. Newman MF, Grocott HP, Mathew JP, et al; Neurologic Outcome Research Group and the Cardiothoracic Anesthesia Research Endeavors (CARE) Investigators of the Duke Heart Center. Report of the substudy assessing the impact of neurocognitive function on quality of life 5 years after cardiac surgery. *Stroke*. 2001;32:2874-2881.

214. McKhann GM, Grega MA, Borowicz LM Jr, et al. Encephalopathy and stroke after coronary artery bypass grafting: incidence, consequences, and prediction. *Arch Neurol*. 2002;59:1422-1428.

215. Selnes OA, Grega MA, Borowicz LM Jr, Royall RM, McKhann GM, Baumgartner WA. Cognitive changes with coronary artery disease: a prospective study of coronary artery bypass graft patients and nonsurgical controls. *Ann Thorac Surg*. 2003;75:1377-1384.

216. Stygall J, Newman SP, Fitzgerald G, et al. Cognitive change 5 years after coronary artery bypass surgery. *Health Psychol*. 2003;22:579-586.

217. Friedland RP, Fritsch T, Smyth KA, et al. Patients with Alzheimer's disease have reduced activities in midlife compared with healthy control-group members. *Proc Natl Acad Sci* (U S A). 2001;98:3440-3445.

218. Verghese L, Lipton RB, Katz MJ, et al. Leisure activities and the risk of dementia in the elderly. *N Engl J Med*. 2003;348:2508-2516.

219. Wilson RS, Barnes LL, Mendes de Leon CF, et al. Depressive symptoms, cognitive decline, and risk of AD in older persons. *Neurology.* 2002;59:364-370.

220. Green RC, Cupples LA, Kurz A, et al. Depression as a risk factor for Alzheimer disease: the MIRAGE Study. *Arch Neurol.* 2003;60:753-759.

221. Wilson RS, Evans DA, Bienias JL, Mendes de Leon CF, Schneider JA, Bennett DA. Proneness to psychological distress is associated with risk of Alzheimer's disease. *Neurology.* 2003;61:1479-1485.

222. Abbott RD, White LR, Ross GW, Masaki KH, Curb JD, Petrovitch H. Walking and dementia in physically capable elderly men. *JAMA.* 2004;292:1447-1453.

223. Weuve J, Kang JH, Manson JE, Breteler MM, Ware JH, Grodstein F. Physical activity, including walking, and cognitive function in older women. *JAMA.* 2004;292:1454-1461.

224. Morris MC, Beckett LA, Scherr PA, et al. Vitamin E and vitamin C supplement use and risk of incident Alzheimer disease. *Alzheimer Dis Assoc Disord.* 1998;12:121-126.

225. Solfrizzi V, Panza F, Torres F, et al. High monounsaturated fatty acids intake protects against age-related cognitive decline. *Neurology.* 1999;52:1563-1569.

226. Engelhart MJ, Geerlings MI, Ruitenberg A, et al. Dietary intake of antioxidants and risk of Alzheimer disease. *JAMA.* 2002;287:3223-3229.

227. Luchsinger JA, Tang MX, Siddiqui M, Shea S, Mayeux R. Alcohol intake and risk of dementia. *J Am Geriatr Soc.* 2004;52:540-546.

228. Luchsinger JA, Tang MX, Shea S, Mayeux R. Caloric intake and the risk of Alzheimer disease. *Arch Neurol.* 2002;59:1258-1263.

229. Morris MC, Evans DA, Bienias JL, et al. Dietary intake of antioxidant nutrients and the risk of incident Alzheimer disease in a biracial community study. *JAMA.* 2002;287:3230-3237.

230. Seshadri S, Wolf PA, Beiser A, et al. Elevated plasma homocysteine levels are associated with subclinical brain injury in healthy adults: Relation to silent cerebral infarcts, white matter hyperintensity and MRI brain volume in the Framingham offspring. *Neurology.* 2003;60:A80.

231. Luchsinger JA, Tang MX, Shea S, Miller J, Green R, Mayeux R. Plasma homocysteine levels and risk of Alzheimer disease. *Neurology.* 2004;62:1972-1976.

232. Levy-Lahad E, Bird TD. Genetic factors in Alzheimer's disease: a review of recent advances. *Ann Neurol.* 1996;40:829-840.

233. Blacker D, Tanzi RE. The genetics of Alzheimer disease: current status and future prospects. *Arch Neurol.* 1998;55:294-296.

234. Janssen JC, Beck JA, Campbell TA, et al. Early onset familial Alzheimer's disease: Mutation frequency in 31 families. *Neurology.* 2003;60:235-239.

235. Rogaeva E, Bergeron C, Sato C, et al. PS1 Alzheimer's disease family with spastic paraplegia: the search for a gene modifier. *Neurology.* 2003;61:1005-1007.

236. Strittmatter WJ, Weisgraber KH, Huang DY, et al. Binding of human apolipoprotein E to synthetic amyloid beta peptide: isoform-specific effects and implications for late-onset Alzheimer's disease. *Proc Natl Acad Sci USA.* 1993;90:8098-8102.

12

237. Rebeck GW, Reiter JS, Strickland DK, Hyman BT. Apolipoprotein E in sporadic Alzheimer's disease: allelic variation and receptor interactions. *Neuron.* 1993;11:575-580.

238. Strittmatter WJ, Weisgraber KH, Goedert M, et al. Hypothesis: microtubule instability and paired helical filament formation in Alzheimer disease brain are related to apolipoprotein E genotype. *Exp Neurol.* 1994;125:163-171; discussion 172-174.

239. Goldgaber D, Schwarzman AI, Bhasin R, et al. Sequestration of amyloid beta-peptide. *Ann NY Acad Sci.* 1993;695:139-143.

240. Roses AD. Apolipoprotein E affects the rate of Alzheimer disease expression: beta-amyloid burden is a secondary consequence dependent on APOE genotype and duration of disease. *J Neuropathol Exp Neurol.* 1994;53:429-437.

241. Strittmatter WJ, Saunders AM, Schmechel D, et al. Apolipoprotein E: high-avidity binding to beta-amyloid and increased frequency of type 4 allele in late-onset familial Alzheimer's disease. *Proc Natl Acad Sci USA.* 1993;90:1977-1981.

242. Saunders AM, Strittmatter WJ, Schmechel D, et al. Association of apolipoprotein E allele ε4 with late-onset familial and sporadic Alzheimer's disease. *Neurology.* 1993;43:1467-1472.

243. Nalbantoglu J, Gilfix BM, Bertrand P, et al. Predictive value of apolipoprotein E genotyping in Alzheimer's disease: results of an autopsy series and an analysis of several combined studies. *Ann Neurol.* 1994;36:889-895.

244. Corder EH, Saunders AM, Strittmatter WJ, et al. Gene dose of apolipoprotein E type 4 allele and the risk of Alzheimer's disease in late onset families. *Science.* 1993;261:921-923.

245. Petersen RC, Smith GE, Ivnik RJ, et al. Apolipoprotein E status as a predictor of the development of Alzheimer's disease in memory-impaired individuals. *JAMA.* 1995;273:1274-1278.

246. Green RC, Stewart W. APOE and the diagnosis of Alzheimer's disease. *Neurology Network Commentary.* 1998;2:191-196.

247. Green RC. Risk assessment for Alzheimer's disease with genetic susceptibility testing: Has the moment arrived? *Alzheimer's Care Quarterly.* 2002;3:208-214.

248. Roberts JS, Connell CM, Cisewski D, Hipps YG, Demissie S, Green RC. Differences between African Americans and whites in their perceptions of Alzheimer disease. *Alzheimer Dis Assoc Disord.* 2003;17:19-26.

249. Roberts JS, LaRusse SA, Katzen H, et al. Reasons for seeking genetic susceptibility testing among first-degree relatives of people with Alzheimer disease. *Alzheimer Dis Assoc Disord.* 2003;17:86-93.

250. Roberts JS, Barber M, Brown TM, et al. Who seeks genetic susceptibility testing for Alzheimer's disease? Findings from a multisite, randomized clinical trial. *Genet Med.* 2004;6:197-203.

251. LaRusse SA, Roberts JS, Monteau T, et al. Genetic susceptibility testing versus family history-based risk assessment : impact on perceived risk of Alzheimer's disease. *Genetics in Medicine.* 2005. In press.

252. Marteau T, Roberts JS, LaRusse SA, et al. Predictive genetic testing for Alzheimer's disease : Impact upon risk perception. *Risk Analysis.* 2005. In press.

253. Zick CD, Matthews C, Zick M, Roberts JS. Genetic susceptibility testing for Alzheimer's disease and its impact on insurance behavior. *Health Affairs.* 2005. In press.

254. Blacker D, Wilcox MA, Laird NM, et al. Alpha-2 macroglobulin is genetically associated with Alzheimer disease. *Nat Genet.* 1998;19: 357-360.

255. Korovaitseva GI, Premkumar S, Grigorenko A, et al. Alpha-2 macroglobulin gene in early- and late-onset Alzheimer disease. *Neurosci Lett.* 1999;271:129-131.

256. Tanzi R. The search for novel Alzheimer's disease genes. *Neurobiol Aging.* 2002;23:S10.

257. Zappia M, Manna I, Serra P, et al. Increased risk for Alzheimer disease with the interaction of MPO and A2M polymorphisms. *Arch Neurol.* 2004;61:341-344.

258. Morris HH 3d, Dinner DS, Luders H, Wyllie E, Kramer R. Supplementary motor seizures: clinical and electroencephalographic findings. *Neurology.* 1988;38:1075-1082.

259. Mendez MF, Mastri AR, Sung JH, Frey WH 2d. Clinically diagnosed Alzheimer disease: neuropathologic findings in 650 cases. *Alzheimer Dis Assoc Disord.* 1992;6:35-43.

260. Becker JT, Boller F, Lopez OL, Saxton J, McGonigle KL. The natural history of Alzheimer's disease. Description of study cohort and accuracy of diagnosis. *Arch Neurol.* 1994;51:585-594.

261. Mayeux R, Saunders AM, Shea S, et al. Utility of the apolipoprotein E genotype in the diagnosis of Alzheimer's disease. Alzheimer's Disease Centers Consortium on Apolipoprotein E and Alzheimer's Disease [published correction appears in *N Engl J Med.* 1998;338: 1325]. *N Engl J Med.* 1998;338:506-511.

262. Salmon DP, Thomas RG, Pay MM, et al. Alzheimer's disease can be accurately diagnosed in very mildly impaired individuals. *Neurology.* 2002;59:1022-1028.

263. McKhann G, Drachman D, Folstein M, Katzman R, Price D, Stadlan EM. Clinical diagnosis of Alzheimer's disease: report of the NINCDS-ADRDA work group. *Neurology.* 1984;34:939-944.

264. Motter R, Vigo-Pelfrey C, Kholodenko D, et al. Reduction of beta-amyloid peptide$_{42}$ in the cerebrospinal fluid of patients with Alzheimer's disease. *Ann Neurol.* 1995;38:643-648.

265. Galasko D, Chang L, Motter R, et al. High cerebrospinal fluid tau and low amyloid beta42 levels in the clinical diagnosis of Alzheimer disease and relation to apolipoprotein E genotype. *Arch Neurol.* 1998;55:937-945.

266. Clark CM, Xie S, Chittams J, et al. Cerebrospinal fluid tau and beta-amyloid: how well do these biomarkers reflect autopsy-confirmed dementia diagnoses? *Arch Neurol.* 2003;60:1696-1702.

267. Sunderland T, Linker G, Mirza N, et al. Decreased beta-amyloid1-42 and increased tau levels in cerebrospinal fluid of patients with Alzheimer disease. *JAMA.* 2003;;289:2094-2103.

268. Ghanbari HA, Miller BE, Haigler HJ, et al. Biochemical assay of Alzheimer's disease—associated protein(s) in human brain tissue. A clinical study. *JAMA.* 1990;263:2907-2910.

269. Ghanbari H, Ghanbari K, Munzar M, Averback P. Specificity of AD7C-NTP as a biochemical marker for Alzheimer's disease. *Contemporary Neurology.* 1998;1998:2-6.

12

270. Ghanbari H, Ghanbari K, Beheshti I, Munzar M, Vasauskas A, Averback P. Biochemical assay for AD7C-NTP in urine as an Alzheimer's disease marker. *J Clin Lab Anal*. 1998;12:285-288.

271. Fukumoto H, Tennis M, Locascio JJ, Hyman BT, Growdon JH, Irizarry MC. Age but not diagnosis is the main predictor of plasma amyloid beta-protein levels. *Arch Neurol*. 2003;60:958-964.

272. Mayeux R, Honig LS, Tang MX, et al. Plasma A[beta]40 and A[beta]42 and Alzheimer's disease: relation to age, mortality, and risk. *Neurology*. 2003;61:1185-1190.

273. Riemenschneider M, Lautenschlager N, Wagenpfeil S, Diehl J, Drzezga A, Kurz A. Cerebrospinal fluid tau and beta-amyloid 42 proteins identify Alzheimer disease in subjects with mild cognitive impairment. *Arch Neurol*. 2002;59:1729-1734.

274. Talamo B, Feng WH, Perez-Cruet L, et al. Pathologic changes in olfactory neurons in Alzheimer's disease. *Ann NY Acad Sci*. 1991;640: 1-7.

275. Etcheberrigaray R, Ito E, Oka K, et al. Potassium channel dysfunction in fibroblasts identifies patients with Alzheimer disease. *Proc Natl Acad Sci USA*. 1993;90:8209-8213.

276. Govoni S, Bergamaschi S, Racchi M, et al. Cytosol protein kinase C downregulation in fibroblasts from Alzheimer's disease patients. *Neurology*. 1993;43:2581-2586.

277. Zubenko GS, Cohen BM, Growdon J, Corkin S. Cell membrane abnormality in Alzheimer's disease. *Lancet*. 1984;2:235. Letter.

278. Zubenko GS, Teply J, Winwood E, et al. Prospective study of increased platelet membrane fluidity as a risk factor for Alzheimer's disease: results at 5 years. *Am J Psychiatry*. 1996;153:420-423.

279. Kennard ML, Feldman H, Yamada T, Jeffries WA. Serum levels of the iron binding protein p97 are elevated in Alzheimer's disease. *Nat Med*. 1996;2:1230-1235.

280. Padovani A, Pastorino L, Borroni B, et al. Amyloid precursor protein in platelets: a peripheral marker for the diagnosis of sporadic AD. *Neurology*. 2001;57:2243-2248.

281. Borroni B, Colciaghi F, Corsini P, et al. Early stages of probable Alzheimer disease are associated with changes inplatelet amyloid precursor protein forms. *Neurol Sci*. 2002;23:207-210.

282. Borroni B, Colciaghi F, Caltagirone C, et al. Platelet amyloid precursor protein abnormalities in mild cognitive impairment predict conversion to dementia of Alzheimer type: a 2-year follow-up study. *Arch Neurol*. 2003;60:1740-1744.

283. Atiya M, Hyman BT, Albert MS, Killiany R. Structural magnetic resonance imaging in established and prodromal Alzheimer disease: a review. *Alzheimer Dis Assoc Disord*. 2003;17:177-195.

284. Jack CR Jr, Petersen RC, Xu YC, et al. Prediction of AD with MRI-based hippocampal volume in mild cognitive impairment. *Neurology*. 1999;52:1397-1403.

285. Gosche KM, Mortimer JA, Smith CD, Markesbery WR, Snowdon DA. Hippocampal volume as an index of Alzheimer neuropathology: findings from the Nun Study. *Neurology*. 2002;58:1476-1482.

286. Du AT, Schuff N, Zhu XP, et al. Atrophy rates of entorhinal cortex in AD and normal aging. *Neurology*. 2003;60:481-486.

287. Jack CR Jr, Slomkowski M, Gracon S, et al. MRI as a biomarker of disease progression in a therapeutic trial of milameline for AD. *Neurology*. 2003;60:253-260.

288. Silbert LC, Quinn JF, Moore MM, et al. Changes in premorbid brain volume predict Alzheimer's disease pathology. *Neurology.* 2003;61: 487-492.

289. Dickerson BC, Salat DH, Bates JF, et al. Medial temporal lobe function and structure in mild cognitive impairment. *Ann Neurol.* 2004;56:27-35.

290. Blennow K. CSF biomarkers for mild cognitive impairment. *J Intern Med.* 2004;256:224-234.

291. Khachaturian Z. The five-five, ten-ten plan for Alzheimer's disease. *Neurobiol Aging.* 1992;13:197-198; discussion 199. Editorial.

292. Annas GJ. Privacy rules for DNA databanks. Protecting coded 'future diaries'. *JAMA.* 1993;270:2346-2350.

293. Harper PS. Research samples from families with genetic diseases: a proposed code of conduct. *BMJ.* 1993;306:1391-1394.

294. Post SG. Genetics, ethics, and Alzheimer disease. *J Am Geriatr Soc.* 1994;42:782-786.

295. Pokorski RJ. Insurance underwriting in the genetic era. *Am J Human Genet.* 1997;60:205-216.

296. Morris JC, Edland S, Clark C, et al. The consortium to establish a registry for Alzheimer's disease (CERAD). Part IV. Rates of cognitive change in the longitudinal assessment of probable Alzheimer's disease. *Neurology.* 1993;43:2457-2465.

297. Stern RG, Mohs RC, Davidson M, et al. A longitudinal study of Alzheimer's disease: measurement, rate, and predictors of cognitive deterioration. *Am J Psychiatry.* 1994;151:390-396.

298. Stern Y, Mayeux R, Sano M, Hauser WA, Bush T. Predictors of disease course in patients with probable Alzheimer's disease. *Neurology.* 1987;37:1649-1653.

299. Morris JC, Drazner M, Fulling K, Grant EA, Goldring J. Clinical and pathological aspects of parkinsonism in Alzheimer's disease. A role for extranigral factors? *Arch Neurol.* 1989;46:651-657.

300. Miller TP, Tinklenberg JR, Brooks JO 3d, Yesavage JA. Cognitive decline in patients with Alzheimer disease: differences in patients with and without extrapyramidal signs. *Alzheimer Dis Assoc Disord.* 1991;5:251-256.

301. Mortimer JA, Ebbitt B, Jun SP, Finch MD. Predictors of cognitive and functional progression in patients with probable Alzheimer's disease. *Neurology.* 1992;42:1689-1696.

302. Chui HC, Lyness SA, Sobel E, Schneider LS. Extrapyramidal signs and psychiatric symptoms predict faster cognitive decline in Alzheimer's disease. *Arch Neurol.* 1994;51:676-681.

303. Miller TP, Tinklenberg JR, Brooks JO 3d, Fenn HH, Yesavage JA. Selected psychiatric symptoms associated with rate of cognitive decline in patients with Alzheimer's disease. *J Geriatr Psychiatry Neurol.* 1993;6:235-238.

304. Yesavage JA, Brooks JO 3d, Taylor J, Tinklenberg J. Development of aphasia, apraxia, and agnosia and decline in Alzheimer's disease. *Am J Psychiatry.* 1993;150:742-747.

305. Haupt M, Pollmann S, Kurz A. Symptom progression in Alzheimer's disease: relation to onset age and familial aggregation. *Acta Neurol Scand.* 1993;88:349-353.

306. Seltzer B, Sherwin I. A comparison of clinical features in early- and late-onset primary degenerative dementia. One entity or two? *Arch Neurol.* 1983;40:143-146.

12

307. Heyman A, Wilkinson WE, Hurwitz BJ, et al. Early-onset Alzheimer's disease: clinical predictors of institutionalization and death. *Neurology.* 1987;37:980-984.

308. Heston LL, Mastri AR, Anderson VE, White J. Dementia of the Alzheimer type. Clinical genetics, natural history, and associated conditions. *Arch Gen Psychiatry.* 1981;38:1085-1090.

309. Knesevich JW, Toro FR, Morris JC, LaBarge E. Aphasia, family history, and the longitudinal course of senile dementia of the Alzheimer type. *Psychiatry Res.* 1985;14:255-263.

310. Huff FJ, Growdon JH, Corkin S, Rosen JT. Age at onset and rate of progression of Alzheimer's disease. *J Am Geriatr Soc.* 1987;35:27-30.

311. Boller F, Becker JT, Holland AL, Forbes MM, Hood PC, McGonigle-Gibson KL. Predictors of decline in Alzheimer's disease. *Cortex.* 1991;27:9-17.

312. Flicker C, Ferris SH, Reisberg B. A longitudinal study of cognitive function in elderly persons with subjective memory complaints. *J Am Geriatr Soc.* 1993;41:1029-1032.

313. Faber-Langendoen K, Morris JC, Knesevich JW, LaBarge E, Miller JP, Berg L. Aphasia in senile dementia of the Alzheimer type. *Ann Neurol.* 1988;23:365-370.

314. Jacobs D, Sano M, Marder K, et al. Age at onset of Alzheimer's disease: relation to pattern of cognitive dysfunction and rate of decline. *Neurology.* 1994;44:1215-1220.

315. Bracco L, Gallato R, Grigoletto F, et al. Factors affecting course and survival in Alzheimer's disease. A 9-year longitudinal study. *Arch Neurol.* 1994;51:1213-1219.

316. Benson DF, Davis RJ, Snyder BD. Posterior cortical atrophy. *Arch Neurol.* 1988;45:789-793.

317. Cogan DG. Visual disturbances with focal progressive dementing disease. *Am J Ophthalmol.* 1985;100:68-72.

318. Crystal HA, Horoupian DS, Katzman R, Jotkowitz S. Biopsy-proved Alzheimer disease presenting as a right parietal lobe syndrome. *Ann Neurol.* 1982;12:186-188.

319. Kirshner HS, Webb WG, Kelly MP, Wells CE. Language disturbance. An initial symptom of cortical degenerations and dementia. *Arch Neurol.* 1984;41:491-496.

320. Martin A, Brouwers P, Lalonde F, et al. Towards a behavioral typology of Alzheimer's patients. *J Clin Exp Neuropsychol.* 1986;8: 594-610.

321. Hof PR, Bouras C, Constantinidis J, Morrison JH. Balint's syndrome in Alzheimer's disease: specific disruption of the occipito-parietal visual pathway. *Brain Res.* 1989;493:368-375.

322. Jagust WJ, Davies P, Tiller-Borich JK, Redd BR. Focal Alzheimer's disease. *Neurology.* 1990;40:14-19.

323. Becker JT, Lopez OL, Wess J. Material-specific memory loss in probable Alzheimer's disease. *J Neurol Neurosurg Psychiatry.* 1992;55: 1177-1181.

324. Mesulam MM. Slowly progressive aphasia without generalized dementia. *Ann Neurol.* 1982;11:592-598.

325. Chawluk JB, Mesulam MM, Hurtig H, et al. Slowly progressive aphasia without generalized dementia: studies with positron emission tomography. *Ann Neurol.* 1986;19:68-74.

326. Weintraub S, Rubin NP, Mesulam MM. Primary progressive aphasia. Longitudinal course, neuropsychological profile, and language features. *Arch Neurol.* 1990;47:1329-1335.

327. Kirshner HS, Tanridag O, Thurman L, Whetsell WO Jr. Progressive aphasia without dementia: two cases with focal spongiform degeneration. *Ann Neurol.* 1987;22:527-532.

328. Green J, Morris JC, Sandson J, McKeel DW Jr, Miller JW. Progressive aphasia: a precursor of global dementia? *Neurology.* 1990;40: 423-429.

329. Feher EP, Doody RS, Whitehead J, Pirozzolo FJ. Progressive nonfluent aphasia with dementia: a case report. *J Geriatr Psychiatry Neurol.* 1991;4:236-240.

330. Kertesz A, Hudson L, Mackenzie IR, Munoz DG. The pathology and nosology of primary progressive aphasia. *Neurology.* 1994; 44:2065-2072.

331. De Renzi E. Slowly progressive visual agnosia or apraxia without dementia. *Cortex.* 1986;22:171-180.

332. Dick JP, Snowden JS, Northen B, Goulding PJ. Slowly progressive apraxia. *Behav Neurol.* 1989;2:101-114.

333. Rapcsak SZ, Ochipa C, Roeltgen MG, Roeltgen DP. Posterior cortical atrophy: neuropsychological and neuroradiological correlates. *Ann Neurol.* 1990;28:255.

334. Okuda B, Tachibana H, Kawabata K, Takeda M, Sugita M. Slowly progressive limb-kinetic apraxia with a decrease in unilateral cerebral blood flow. *Acta Neurol Scand.* 1992;86:76-81.

335. Azouvi P, Bergego C, Robel L, et al. Slowly progressive apraxia: two case studies. *J Neurol.* 1993;240:347-350.

336. Pollmann S, Haupt M, Romero B, Kurz A. Stability of cognitive symptoms in dementia of the Alzheimer type. *Dementia.* 1992;3:328-334.

337. Beatty WW, Winn P, Adams RL, et al. Preserved cognitive skills in dementia of the Alzheimer type. *Arch Neurol.* 1994;51:1040-1046.

338. Molsa PK, Marttila RJ, Rinne UK. Extrapyramidal signs in Alzheimer's disease. *Neurology.* 1984;34:1114-1116.

339. Chui HC, Teng EL, Henderson VW, Moy AC. Clinical subtypes of dementia of the Alzheimer type. *Neurology.* 1985;35:1544-1550.

340. Mayeux R, Stern Y, Spanton S. Heterogeneity in the dementia of the Alzheimer type: evidence of subgroups. *Neurology.* 1985;35:453-461.

341. Funkenstein HH, Albert MS, Cook NR, et al. Extrapyramidal signs and other neurologic findings in clinically diagnosed Alzheimer's disease. A community-based study. *Arch Neurol.* 1993;50:51-56.

342. Leverenz J, Sumi SM. Parkinson's disease in patients with Alzheimer's disease. *Arch Neurol.* 1986;43:662-664.

343. Soininen H, Laulumaa V, Helkala EL, Hartikainen P, Riekkinen PJ. Extrapyramidal signs in Alzheimer's disease: a 3-year follow-up study. *J Neural Transm Park Dis Dement Sect.* 1992;4:107-119.

344. Merello M, Sabe L, Teson A, et al. Extrapyramidalism in Alzheimer's disease: prevalence, psychiatric, and neuropsychological correlates. *J Neurol Neurosurg Psychiatry.* 1994;57:1503-1509.

345. Haan MN, Jagust WJ, Galasko D, Kaye J. Effect of extrapyramidal signs and Lewy bodies on survival in patients with Alzheimer disease. *Arch Neurol.* 2002;59:588-593.

346. Basavaraju NG, Silverstone FA, Libaow LS, Paraskevas K. Primitive reflexes and perceptual sensory tests in the elderly—their usefulness in dementia. *J Chronic Dis.* 1981;34:367-377.

12

347. Franssen EH, Reisberg B, Kluger A, Sinaiko E, Boja C. Cognition-independent neurologic symptoms in normal aging and probable Alzheimer's disease. *Arch Neurol.* 1991;48:148-154.

348. Richards M, Stern Y, Mayeux R. Subtle extrapyramidal signs can predict the development of dementia in elderly individuals. *Neurology.* 1993;43:2184-2188.

349. Galasko D, Kwo-on-Yuen PF, Klauber MR, Thal L. Neurological findings in Alzheimer's disease and normal aging. *Arch Neurol.* 1990;47:625-627.

350. Franssen EH, Kluger A, Torossian CL, Reisberg B. The neurologic syndrome of severe Alzheimer's disease. Relationship to functional decline. *Arch Neurol.* 1993;50:1029-1039.

351. Mayeux R, Albert M, Jenike M. Physostigmine-induced myoclonus in Alzheimer's disease. *Neurology.* 1987;37:345-346.

352. Forstl H, Burns A, Levy R, Cairns N, Luthert P, Lantos P. Neurologic signs in Alzheimer's disease. Results of a prospective clinical and neuropathologic study. *Arch Neurol.* 1992;49:1038-1042.

353. Wilson RS, Beckett LA, Barnes LL, et al. Individual differences in rates of change in cognitive abilities of older persons. *Psychol Aging.* 2002;17:179-193.

354. Howieson DB, Camicioli R, Quinn J, et al. Natural history of cognitive decline in the old old. *Neurology.* 2003;60:1489-1494.

355. Bolla KI, Lindgren KN, Bonaccorsy C, Bleecker ML. Memory complaints in older adults. Fact or fiction? *Arch Neurol.* 1991;48:61-64.

356. Gagnon M, Dartigues JF, Mazaux JM, et al. Self-reported memory complaints and memory performance in elderly French community residents: results of the PAQUID Research Program. *Neuroepidemiology.* 1994;13:145-154.

357. Troster AI, Moe KE, Vitiello MV, Prinz PN. Predicting long-term outcome in individuals at risk for Alzheimer's disease with the Dementia Rating Scale. *J Neuropsychiatry Clin Neurosci.* 1994;6:54-57.

358. Kawas CH, Corrada MM, Brookmeyer R, et al. Visual memory predicts Alzheimer's disease more than a decade before diagnosis. *Neurology.* 2003;60:1089-1093.

359. Petersen RC, Stevens JC, Ganguli M, Tangalos EG, Cummings JL, DeKosky ST. Practice parameter: early detection of dementia: mild cognitive impairment (an evidence-based review). Report of the Quality Standards Subcommittee of the American Academy of Neurology. *Neurology.* 2001;56:1133-1142.

360. Bennett DA. Mild cognitive impairment. *Clin Geriatr Med.* 2004;20:15-25.

361. Petersen RC. Mild cognitive impairment as a diagnostic entity. *J Intern Med.* 2004;256:183-194.

362. Petersen RC. Normal aging, mild cognitive impairment, and early Alzheimer's disease. *The Neurologist.* 1995;1:326-344.

363. Rubin EH, Morris JC, Grant EA, Vendegna T. Very mild senile dementia of the Alzheimer type. I. Clinical assessment. *Arch Neurol.* 1989;46:379-382.

364. Flicker C, Ferris SH, Reisberg B. Mild cognitive impairment in the elderly: predictors of dementia. *Neurology.* 1991;41:1006-1009.

365. Morris JC, McKeel DW Jr, Storandt M, et al. Very mild Alzheimer's disease: informant based clinical, psychometric, and pathologic distinction from normal aging. *Neurology.* 1991;41:469-478.

366. Dawe B, Procter A, Phlpot M. Concepts of mild memory impairment in the elderly and their relationship to dementia: A review. *Int J Geriatr Psychiatry*. 1992;7:473-479.

367. Jacobs DM, Sano M, Dooneief G, Marder K, Bell KL, Stern Y. Neuropsychological detection and characterization of preclinical Alzheimer's disease. *Neurology*. 1995;45:957-962.

368. Linn RT, Wolf PA, Bachman DL, et al. The 'preclinical phase' of probable Alzheimer's disease. A 13-year prospective study of Framingham cohort. *Arch Neurol*. 1995;52:485-490.

369. Tuokko H, Frerichs R, Graham J, et al. Five-year follow-up of cognitive impairment with no dementia. *Arch Neurol*. 2003;60:577-582.

370. Bowen J, Teri L, Kukull W, McCormick W, McCurry SM, Larson EB. Progression of dementia in patients with isolated memory loss. *Lancet*. 1997;349:763-765.

371. Bruscoli M, Lovestone S. Is MCI really just early dementia? A systematic review of conversion studies. *Int Psychogeriatr*. 2004;16:129-140.

372. Chetelat G, Desgranges B, de la Sayette V, Viader F, Eustache F, Baron JC. Mild cognitive impairment: Can FDG-PET predict who is to rapidly convert to Alzheimer's disease? *Neurology*. 2003;60:1374-1377.

373. Tervo S, Kivipelto M, Hanninen T, et al. Incidence and risk factors for mild cognitive impairment: a population-based three-year follow-up study of cognitively healthy elderly subjects. *Dement Geriatr Cogn Disord*. 2004;17:196-203.

374. Wolf H, Ecke GM, Bettin S, Dietrich J, Gertz HJ. Do white matter changes contribute to the subsequent development of dementia in patients with mild cognitive impairment? A longitudinal study. *Int J Geriatr Psychiatry*. 2000;15:803-812.

375. Tabert MH, Albert SM, Borukhova-Milov L, et al. Functional deficits in patients with mild cognitive impairment: prediction of AD. *Neurology*. 2002;58:758-764.

376. Morris JC, Storandt M, Miller JP, et al. Mild cognitive impairment represents early-stage Alzheimer disease. *Arch Neurol*. 2001;58:397-405.

377. Hwang TJ, Masterman DL, Ortiz F, Fairbanks LA, Cummings JL. Mild cognitive impairment is associated with characteristic neuropsychiatric symptoms. *Alzheimer Dis Assoc Disord*. 2004;18:17-21.

378. Grundman M, Petersen RC, Ferris SH, et al; Alzheimer's Disease Cooperative Study. Mild cognitive impairment can be distinguished from Alzheimer disease and normal aging for clinical trials. *Arch Neurol*. 2004;61:59-66.

379. Bullock R, Hammond G. Realistic expectations: the management of severe Alzheimer disease. *Alzheimer Dis Assoc Disord*. 2003;17(suppl 3):S80-S85.

380. Hui JS, Wilson RS, Bennett DA, Bienias JL, Gilley DW, Evans DA. Rate of cognitive decline and mortality in Alzheimer's disease. *Neurology*. 2003;61:1356-1361.

381. Wolfson C, Wolfson DB, Asgharian M, et al; Clinical Progression of Dementia Study Group. A reevaluation of the duration of survival after the onset of dementia. *N Engl J Med*. 2001;344:1111-1116.

382. Post SG, Whitehouse PJ. The moral basis for limiting treatment: hospice care and advanced progressive dementia. In: Volicer L, Hurley

A, eds. *Hospice Care for Patients with Advanced Progressive Dementia.* New York, NY: Springer; 1998:117-131.

383. Volicer L, Hurley A. *Hospice Care for Patients with Advanced Progressive Dementia.* New York, NY: Springer; 1998.

384. Terry RD, Katzman R. Senile dementia of the Alzheimer type: defining a disease. In: Katzman R, eds. *Neurology of Aging.* Philadelphia, Pa: FA Davis; 1983:51-84.

385. Mann DM. The topographic distribution of brain atrophy in Alzheimer's disease. *Acta Neuropathol.* 1991;83:81-86.

386. Kidd M. Paired helical filaments in electron microscopy in Alzheimer's disease. *Nature.* 1963;197:192-193.

387. Terry RD. The fine structure of neurofibrillary tangles in Alzheimer's disease. *J Neuropathol Exp Neurol.* 1963;22:629-642.

388. Terry RD. Aging senile dementia. In: Katzman R, Terry RD, Bick KL, eds. *Alzheimer's Disease: Senile Dementia and Related Disorders.* New York, NY: Raven Press; 1978:11.

389. Lee VM, Balin BJ, Otvos L Jr, Trojanowski JQ. A68: A major subunit of paired helical filaments and derivatized forms of normal tau. *Science.* 1991;251:675-678.

390. Hof P, Morrison JH. The cellular basis of cortical disconnection in Alzheimer disease and related dementing conditions. In: Terry RD, Katzman R, Bick KL, eds. *Alzheimer Disease.* New York, NY: Raven Press; 1994.

391. Iqbal K, Alonso Adel C, El-Akkad E, et al. Alzheimer neurofibrillary degeneration: therapeutic targets and high-throughput assays. *J Mol Neurosci.* 2003;20:425-429.

392. Selkoe DJ. Alzheimer's disease: a central role for amyloid. *J Neuropathol Exp Neurol.* 1994;53:438-447.

393. Selkoe DJ. Alzheimer's disease: genotypes, phenotype, and treatments. *Science.* 1997;275:630-631.

394. Hardy J, Selkoe DJ. The amyloid hypothesis of Alzheimer's disease: progress and problems on the road to therapeutics. *Science.* 2002;297:353-356.

395. Haass C, Selkoe DJ. Cellular processing of abeta-amyloid precursor protein and the genesis of amyloid beta-peptide. *Cell.* 1993;75:1039-1042.

396. Lambert MP, Barlow AK, Chromy BA, et al. Diffusible, nonfibrillar ligands derived from Abeta1-42 are potent central nervous system neurotoxins. *Proc Natl Acad Sci USA.* 1998;95:6448-6453.

397. Klein WL. Abeta toxicity in Alzheimer's disease: globular oligomers (ADDLs) as new vaccine and drug targets. *Neurochem Int.* 2002;41:345-352.

398. Ingelsson M, Fukumoto H, Newell KL, et al. Early Abeta accumulation and progressive synaptic loss, gliosis, and tangle formation in AD brain. *Neurology.* 2004;62:925-931.

399. Giannakopoulos P, Herrmann FR, Bussiere T, et al. Tangle and neuron numbers, but not amyloid load, predict cognitive status in Alzheimer's disease. *Neurology.* 2003;60:1495-1500.

400. Blocq P, Marinesco G. Sur les lesions et al pathogenie de l'epilepsie dite essentielle. *Sem Med (Paris).* 1892;12:445.

401. Wisniewski HM, Terry RD. Re-examination of the pathogenesis of the senile plaque. *Prog Neuropathol.* 1973;2:1-26.

402. Probst A, Langui D, Ulrich J. Alzheimer's disease: a description of the structural lesions. *Brain Pathol.* 1991;1:229-239.

214

403. Rogers J, Luber-Narod J, Styren SD, Civin WH. Expression of immune system associated antigens by cells of the human central nervous system: relationship to the pathology of Alzheimer's disease. *Neurobiol Aging.* 1988;9:339-349.

404. McGeer PL, McGeer EG. The inflammatory response system of brain: implications for therapy of Alzheimer and other neurodegenerative diseases. *Brain Res Rev.* 1995;21:195-218.

405. Yan SD, Chen X, Fu J, et al. RAGE and amyloid-beta-peptide neurotoxicity in Alzheimer's disease. *Nature.* 1996;382:685-691.

406. Rego AC, Oliveira CR. Mitochondrial dysfunction and reactive oxygen species in excitotoxicity and apoptosis: implications for the pathogenesis of neurodegenerative diseases. *Neurochem Res.* 2003;28:1563-1574.

407. Veurink G, Fuller SJ, Atwood CS, Martins RN. Genetics, lifestyle and the roles of amyloid beta and oxidative stress in Alzheimer's disease. *Ann Hum Biol.* 2003;30:639-667.

408. Davies P, Maloney AJ. Selective loss of central cholinergic neurons in Alzheimer's disease. *Lancet.* 1976;2:1403. Letter.

409. Whitehouse PJ, Price DL, Clark AW, Coyle JT, DeLong MR. Alzheimer disease: evidence for selective loss of cholinergic neurons in the nucleus basalis. *Ann Neurol.* 1981;10:122-126.

410. Bartus RT, Dean RL 3d, Beer B, Lippa AS. The cholinergic hypothesis of geriatric memory dysfunction. *Science.* 1982;217:408-414.

411. Bowen DM, Benton JS, Spillane JA, Smith CC, Allen SJ. Choline acetyltransferase activity and histopathology of frontal neocortex from biopsies of demented patients. *J Neurol Sci.* 1982;57:191-202.

412. Coyle JR, Price DL, DeLong MR. Alzheimer's disease: a disorder of cortical cholinergic innervation. *Science.* 1983;219:1184-1190.

413. Tomlinson BE, Irving D, Blessed G. Cell loss in the locus coeruleus in senile dementia of Alzheimer type. *J Neurol Sci.* 1981;49:419-428.

414. Bondareff W, Mountjoy CQ, Roth M. Loss of neurons of origin of the adrenergic projection to cerebral cortex (nucleus locus coeruleus) in senile dementia. *Neurology.* 1982;32:164-168.

415. Zweig RM, Ross CA, Hedreen JC, et al. The neuropathology of aminergic nuclei in Alzheimer's disease. *Ann Neurol.* 1988;24:233-242.

416. Zarow C, Lyness SA, Mortimer JA, Chui HC. Neuronal loss is greater in the locus coeruleus than nucleus basalis and substantia nigra in Alzheimer and Parkinson diseases. *Arch Neurol.* 2003;60:337-341.

417. Rossor M, Emson P, Dawbarn D, Dockray G, Mountjoy C, Roth M. Postmortem studies of peptides in Alzheimer's disease and Huntington's disease. *Res Publ Assoc Res Nerv Ment Dis.* 1986;64:259-277.

418. Yamamoto T, Hirano A. Nucleus raphe dorsalis in Alzheimer's disease: neurofibrillary tangles and loss of large neurons. *Ann Neurol.* 1985;17:573-577.

419. Deutsch SI, Morihisa JM. Glutamatergic abnormalities in Alzheimer's disease and a rationale for clinical trials with L-glutamate. *Clin Neuropharmacol.* 1988;11:18-35.

420. Proctor AW, Palmer AM, Francis PT, et al. Evidence of glutamatergic denervation and possible abnormal metabolism in Alzheimer's disease. *J Neurochem.* 1988;50:790-802.

421. Davies P. Neurotransmitter-related enzymes in senile dementia of the Alzheimer type. *Brain Res.* 1979;171:319-327.

215

422. Ellison DW, Beal MF, Mazurek MF, Bird ED, Martin JB. A postmortem study of amino acid neurotransmitters in Alzheimer's disease. *Ann Neurol*. 1986;20:616-621.

423. Auchus AP, Green RC, Nemeroff CB. Cortical and subcortical neuropeptides in Alzheimer's disease. *Neurobiol Aging*. 1994;15:589-595.

424. Struble RG, Powers RE, Casanova MF, Kitt CA, Brown EC, Price DL. Neuropeptidergic systems in plaques of Alzheimer's disease. *J Neuropathol Exp Neurol*. 1987;46:567-584.

425. Mesulam MM, Geula C, Moran MA. Anatomy of cholinesterase inhibition in Alzheimer's disease: effect of physostigmine and tetrahydroaminoacridine on plaques and tangles. *Ann Neurol*. 1987;22:683-691.

426. Roberts GW, Crow TJ, Polak JM. Location of neuronal tangles in somatostatin neurons in Alzheimer's disease. *Nature*. 1985;314:92-94.

427. Khachaturian ZS. Diagnosis of Alzheimer's disease. *Arch Neurol*. 1985;42:1097-1105.

428. Paulus W, Bancher C, Jellinger K. Interrater reliability in the neuropathologic diagnosis of Alzheimer's disease. *Neurology*. 1992;42:329-332.

429. Chui HC, Tierney M, Zarow C, Lewis A, Sobel E, Perlmutter LS. Neuropathologic diagnosis of Alzheimer disease: interrater reliability in the assessment of senile plaques and neurofibrillary tangles. *Alzheimer Dis Assoc Disord*. 1993;7:48-54.

430. Wisniewski HM, Robe A, Zigman W, Silverman W. Neuropathological diagnosis of Alzheimer disease. *J Neuropathol Exp Neurol*. 1989;48:606-609.

431. Crystal H, Dickson D, Fuld P, et al. Clinico-pathological studies in dementia: nondemented subjects with pathologically confirmed Alzheimer's disease. *Neurology*. 1988;38:1682-1687.

432. Crystal HA, Dickson DW, Sliwinski MJ, et al. Pathological markers associated with normal aging and dementia in the elderly. *Ann Neurol*. 1993;34:566-573.

433. Markesbery WR. Neuropathological criteria for the diagnosis of Alzheimer's disease. *Neurobiol Aging*. 1997;18(suppl 4):S13-S19.

434. Mirra SS, Heyman A, McKeel D, et al. The Consortium to Establish a Registry for Alzheimer's Disease (CERAD). Part II. Standardization of the neuropathologic assessment of Alzheimer's disease. *Neurology*. 1991;41:479-486.

435. Mirra SS, Gearing M, McKeel DW Jr, et al. Interlaboratory comparison of neuropathology assessments in Alzheimer's disease: a study of the Consortium to Establish a Registry for Alzheimer's Disease (CERAD) [published correction appears in *J Neuropathol Exp Neurol*. 1994;53:425]. *J Neuropathol Exp Neurol*. 1994;53:303-315.

436. Braak H, Braak E. Neuropathological staging of Alzheimer-related changes. *Acta Neuropathol*. 1991;82:239-259.

437. Braak H, Braak E. Pathology of Alzheimer's disease. In: Calne DB, ed. *Neurodegenerative Diseases*. Philadelphia, Pa: WB Saunders; 1994:585-613.

438. Geddes JW, Snowdon DA, Soultanian NS, et al. Braak stages III-IV of Alzheimer-related neuropathology are associated with mild memory loss, stages V-VI are associated with dementia: findings from the Nun Study. *J Neuropathol Exp Neurol*. 1996;55:617.

439. Group NRIW. Consensus recommendations for the postmortem diagnosis of Alzheimer's disease. The National Institute on Aging and Reagan Institute Working Group on Diagnostic Criteria for the Neu-

ropathological Assessment of Alzheimer's Disease. *Neurobiol Aging.* 1997;18(suppl 4):S1-S2.

440. Games D, Adams D, Alessandrini R, et al. Alzheimer-type neuropathology in transgenic mice overexpressing V717F beta-amyloid precursor protein. *Nature.* 1995;373:523-527.

441. Price DL, Becher MW, Wong PC, Borchelt DR, Lee MK, Sisodia SS. Inherited neurodegenerative diseases and transgenic models. *Brain Pathol.* 1996;6:467-480.

442. Irizarry MC, Soriano F, McNamara M, et al. Abeta deposition is associated with neuropil changes, but not with overt neuronal loss in the human amyloid precursor protein V717F(PDAPP) transgeneic mouse. *J Neurosci.* 1997;17:7053-7059.

443. Wyss-Coray T, Masliah E, Mallory M, et al. Amyloidogenic role of cytokine TGF-beta1 in transgenic mice and in Alzheimer's disease. *Nature.* 1997;389:603-606.

444. Borchelt DR, Ratovitski T, van Lare J, et al. Accelerated amyloid deposition in the brains of transgenic mice coexpressing mutant presenilin 1 and amyloid precursor proteins. *Neuron.* 1997;19:939-945.

445. Holcomb L, Gordon MN, McGowan E, et al. Accelerated Alzheimer-type phenotype in transgenic mice carrying both mutant amyloid precursor protein and presenilin 1 transgenes. *Nat Med.* 1998;4:97-100.

446. Bales KR, Verina T, Dodel RC, et al. Lack of apolipoprotein E dramatically reduces amyloid beta-peptide deposition. *Nat Genet.* 1997;17:263-264. Letter.

447. Mittelman MS, Ferris SH, Shulman E, Steinberg G, Levin B. A family intervention to delay nursing home placement of patients with Alzheimer disease. A randomized controlled trial. *JAMA.* 1996;276: 1725-1731.

448. Brown WM. Pharmacotherapy of Alzheimer's disease. *Alzheimer's Disease: Current Treatments and Future Prospects.* London, UK: Financial Times Business, 1999:33-82.

449. Drachman DA. Memory and cognitive function in man: does the cholinergic system have a specific role? *Neurology.* 1977;27:783-790.

450. Petersen RC. Scopolamine state-dependent memory processes in man. *Psychopharmacology.* 1979;64:309-314.

451. McGeer PL, McGeer EG, Suzuki J, Dolman CE, Nagai T. Aging, Alzheimer's disease, and the cholinergic system of the basal forebrain. *Neurology.* 1984;34:741-745.

452. Perry EK, Perry RH. The cholinergic system of Alzheimer disease. In: Roberts P, ed. *Biochemistry of Dementia.* Chichester, UK: John Wiley & Sons; 1980:135.

453. Perry EK. The cholinergic hypothesis—ten years on. *Br Med Bull.* 1986;42:63-69.

454. Mash DC, Flynn DD, Potter LT. Loss of M2 muscarine receptors in the cerebral cortex in Alzheimer's disease and experimental cholinergic denervation. *Science.* 1985;228:1115-1117.

455. DeKosky ST, Harbaugh RE, Schmitt FA, et al. Cortical biopsy in Alzheimer's disease: diagnostic accuracy and neurochemical, neuropathological and cognitive correlations. *Ann Neurol.* 1992;32:625-632.

456. Francis PT, Palmer AM, Sims NR, et al. Neurochemical studies of early-onset Alzheimer's disease. Possible influence on treatment. *N Engl J Med.* 1985;313:7-11.

12

457. Perry EK, Tomlinson BE, Blessed G, Bergmann K, Gibson PH, Perry RH. Correlation of cholinergic abnormalities with senile plaques and mental test scores in senile dementia. *Br Med J.* 1978;2:1457-1459.

458. Rossor MN, Garrett NJ, Johnson AL, Mountjoy CQ, Roth M, Iversen LL. A post-mortem study of the cholinergic and GABA systems in senile dementia. *Brain.* 1982;105:313-330.

459. Growdon JH. Muscarinic agonists in Alzheimer's disease. *Life Sci.* 1997;60:993-998.

460. Bodick NC, Offen WW, Levey AI, et al. Effects of xanomeline, a selective muscarinic receptor antagonist, on cognitive function and behavioral symptoms in Alzheimer disease. *Arch Neurol.* 1997;54:465-473.

461. Kumar R. Efficacy and safety of SB202026. *Ann Neurol.* 1996;40:504.

462. Thal L, Forrest M, Loft H, Mengel H. Lu 25-109, a muscarinic agonist, fails to improve cognition in Alzheimer's disease. LU25-109 Study Group. *Neurology.* 2000;54:421-426.

463. Davis KL, Thal LJ, Gamzu ER, et al. A double-blind, placebo-controlled multicenter study of tacrine for Alzheimer's disease. The Tacrine Collaborative Study Group. *N Engl J Med.* 1992;327:1253-1259.

464. Farlow M, Gracon SI, Hershey LA, Lewis KW, Sadowsky CH, Dolan-Ureno J. A controlled trial of tacrine in Alzheimer's disease. The Tacrine Study Group. *JAMA.* 1992;268:2523-2529.

465. Knapp MJ, Knopman DS, Solomon PR, Pendlebury WW, Davis CS, Gracon SI. A 30-week randomized controlled trial of high-dose tacrine in patients with Alzheimer's disease. The Tacrine Study Group. *JAMA.* 1994;271:985-991.

466. Small GW. Tacrine for treating Alzheimer's disease. *JAMA.* 1992;268:2564-2565. Editorial.

467. Growdon JH. Treatment for Alzheimer's disease? *N Engl J Med.* 1992;327:1306-1308. Editorial.

468. Winker MA. Tacrine for Alzheimer's disease. Which patient, what dose? *JAMA.* 1994;271:1023-1024. Editorial.

469. Schneider LS. Clinical pharmacology of aminoacridines in Alzheimer's disease. *Neurology.* 1993;43(suppl 4):S64-S79.

470. Schneider LS. Tacrine development experience: early clinical trials and enrichment and parallel designs. *Alzheimer Dis Assoc Disord.* 1994;8(suppl 2):S12-S21.

471. Mohs RC, Rosen WG, Davis KL. The Alzheimer's disease assessment scale: an instrument for assessing treatment efficacy. *Psychopharmacol Bull.* 1983;19:448-450.

472. Rosen WG, Mohs RC, Davis KL. A new rating scale for Alzheimer's disease. *Am J Psychiatry.* 1984;141:1356-1364.

473. Clinical Research Working Group for the Pharmaceutical Industry on Dementia. Recommendations for clinical drug trials in dementia. *Dementia.* 1990;1:292-295.

474. Kim YS, Nibbelink DW, Overall JE. Factor structure and reliability of the Alzheimer's Disease Assessment Scale in a multicenter trial with linopirdine. *J Geriatr Psychiatry Neurol.* 1994;7:74-83.

475. Rockwood K. Use of global assessment measures in dementia drug trials. *J Clin Epidemiol.* 1994;47:101-103.

476. Knopman DS, Knapp MJ, Gracon SI, Davis CS. The Clinician Interview-Based Impression (CIBI): a clinician's global change rating scale in Alzheimer's disease. *Neurology.* 1994;44:2315-2321.

477. Cummings JL. Use of cholinesterase inhibitors in clinical practice: evidence-based recommendations. *Am J Geriatr Psychiatry.* 2003;11:131-145.

478. Rogers SL, Friedhoff LT. The efficacy and safety of donepezil in patients with Alzheimer's disease: results of a US multicentre randomized, double-blind, placebo-controlled trial. The Donepezil Study Group. *Dementia.* 1996;7:293-303.

479. Rogers SL, Doody RS, Mohs RC, Friedhoff LT. Donepezil improves cognition and global function in Alzheimer disease: a 15-week, double-blind, placebo-controlled study. Donepezil Study Group. *Arch Intern Med.* 1998;158:1021-1031.

480. Rogers SL, Farlow MR, Doody RS, Mohs R, Friedhoff LT. A 24-week, double-blind, placebo-controlled trial of donepezil in patients with Alzheimer's disease. Donepezil Study Group. *Neurology.* 1998;50:136-145.

481. Winblad B, Engedal K, Soininen H, et al; Donepezil Nordic Study Group. A 1-year, randomized, placebo-controlled study of donepezil in patients with mild to moderate AD. *Neurology.* 2001;57:489-495.

483. Cummings JL, Donohue JA, Brooks RL. The relationship between donepezil and behavioral disturbances in patients with Alzheimer's disease. *Am J Geriatr Psychiatry.* 2000;8:134-140.

482. Mohs RC, Doody RS, Morris JC, et al; "312" Study Group. A 1-year placebo-controlled preservation of function survival study of donepezil in AD patients. *Neurology.* 2001;57:481-488.

484. Feldman H, Gauthier S, Hecker J, Vellas B, Subbiah P, Whalen E; Donepezil MSAD Study Investigators Group. A 24-week, randomized, double-blind study of donepezil in moderate to severe Alzheimer's disease. *Neurology.* 2001;57:613-620.

485. Feldman H, Spiegel R, Quarg P. An evaluation of the effects of rivastigmine on daily function in Alzheimer's disease at different levels of cognitive impairment. *Neurology.* 2003;60:A142.

486. Doody RS, Pratt RD, Persomo CA, Group tDaVS. Donepezil-treated patients demonstrate global benefits on the Clinician's Interview-Based Impression of Change-Plus Version: a comparison of Alzheimer's disease versus vascular dementia. *Neurology.* 2003;60:A412.

487. Aarsland D, Laake K, Larsen JP, Janvin C. Donepezil for cognitive impairment in Parkinson's disease: a randomised controlled study. *J Neurol Neurosurg Psychiatry.* 2002;72:708-712.

488. Leroi I, Brandt J, Reich SG, et al. Randomized placebo-controlled trial of donepezil in cognitive impairment in Parkinson's disease. *Int J Geriatr Psychiatry.* 2004;19:1-8.

489. Salloway S, Ferris S, Kluger A, et al; Donepezil 401 Study Group. Efficacy of donepezil in mild cognitive impairment: a randomized placebo-controlled trial. *Neurology.* 2004;63:651-657.

490. Petersen R, Grundman M, Thomas R, et al. Donepezil and vitamin E as treatments for mild cognitive impairment. *Neurobiol Aging.* 2004;25(suppl 2):20.

491. Grossberg GT, Stahelin HB, Messina JC, Anand R, Veach J. Lack of adverse pharmacodynamic drug interactions with rivastigmine and twenty-two classes of medicaitons. *Int J Geriatr Psychiatry.* 2000;15:242-247.

492. Corey-Bloom J, Anand R, Veach J. A randomized trial evaluating the efficacy and safety of ENA 713 (rivastigmine tartrate), a new acetyl-

cholinesterase inhibitor, in patients with mild to moderately severe Alzheimer's disease. *Int J Geriatr Psychopharmacol.* 1998;1:55-65.

493. Rosler M, Anand R, Cicin-Sain A, et al. Efficacy and safety of rivastigmine in patients with Alzheimer's disease: international randomised controlled trial. *BMJ.* 1999;318:633-638.

494. Kumar V, Anand R, Messina J, Hartman R, Veach J. An efficacy and safety analysis of Exelon in Alzheimer's disease patients with concurrent vascular risk factors. *Eur J Neurology.* 2000. In press.

495. Raskind MA, Peskind ER, Wessel T, Yuan W, the Galantamine USA-Study Group. Galantamine in AD: a 6-month randomized, placebo-controlled trial with a 6-month extension. *Neurology.* 2000;54:2261-2268.

496. Tariot PN, Solomon PR, Morris JC, et al. A 5-month, randomized, placebo-controlled trial of galantamine in AD. *Neurology.* 2000;54:2269-2276.

497. Wilcock GK, Lilienfeld S, Gaens E. Efficacy and safety of galantamine in patients with mild to moderate Alzheimer's disease: multicentre randomised controlled trial. Galantamine International-1 Study Group. *BMJ.* 2000;321:1445-1449.

498. Blesa R, Davidson M, Kurz A, Reichman W, van Baelen B, Schwalen S. Galantamine provides sustained benefits in patients with 'advanced moderate' Alzheimer's disease for at least 12 months. *Dement Geriatr Cogn Disord.* 2003;15:79-87.

499. Aarsland D, Hutchinson M, Larsen JP. Cognitive, psychiatric and motor response to galantamine in Parkinson's disease with dementia. *Int J Geriatr Psychiatry.* 2003;18:937-941.

500. Farlow MR, Cyrus PA. Metrifonate therapy in Alzheimer's disease: a pooled analysis of four randomized, double-blind, placebo-controlled trials. *Dement Geriatr Cogn Disord.* 2000;11:202-211.

501. Zangara A. The psychopharmacology of huperzine A: an alkaloid with cognitive enhancing and neuroprotective properties of interest in the treatment of Alzheimer's disease. *Pharmacol Biochem Behav.* 2003;75:675-686.

502. Farlow MR, Hake A, Messina J, Hartman R, Veach J, Anand R. Response of patients with Alzheimer disease to rivastimine treatment is predicted by the rate of disease progression. *Arch Neurol.* 2001;58:417-422.

503. Farlow M, Ptokin S, Koumaras B, Veach J, Mirski D. Analysis of outcome in retrieved dropout patients in a rivastigmine vs placebo, 26-week Alzheimer disease trial. *Arch Neurol.* 2003;60:843-848.

504. Rogers SL, Friedhoff LT. Long-term efficacy and safety of donepezil in the treatment of Alzheimer's disease: an interim analysis of the results of a US multicentre open label extension study. *Eur Neuropsychopharmacol.* 1998;8:67-75.

505. Doody RS, Geldmacher DS, Gordon B, Perdomo CA, Pratt RD; Donepezil Study Group. Open-label, multicenter, phase 3 extension study of the safety and efficacy of donepezil in patients with Alzheimer disease. *Arch Neurol.* 2001;58:427-433.

506. Trinh NH, Hoblyn J, Mohanty S, Yaffe K. Efficacy of cholinesterase inhibitors in the treatment of neuropsychiatric symptoms and functional impairment in Alzheimer disease: a meta-analysis. *JAMA.* 2003;289:210-216.

507. Rogawski MA, Wenk GL. The neuropharmacological basis for the use of memantine in the treatment of Alzheimer's disease. *CNS Drug Rev.* 2003;9:275-308.

508. Lipton SA, Rosenberg PA. Excitatory amino acids as a final common pathway for neurologic disorders. *N Engl J Med.* 1994;330:613-622.

509. Perry G, Nunomura A, Cash AD, et al. Reactive oxygen: its sources and significance in Alzheimer disease. *J Neural Transm Suppl.* 2002;(62):69-75.

510. Miguel-Hidalgo JJ, Alvarez XA, Cacabelos R, Quack G. Neuroprotection by memantine against neurodegeneration induced by beta-amyloid (1-40). *Brain Res.* 2002;958:210-221.

511. Mattson MP. Antigenic changes similar to those seen in neurofibrillary tangels are elicited by glutamate and Ca^{2+} influx in cultured hippoampal neurons. *Neuron.* 1990;4:105-117.

512. Pizza M, Valerio A, Arrighi V, et al. Inhibition of glutamate-induced neurotoxicity by a tau antisense oligonucleotide in primary culture of rat cerebellar granule cells. *Eur J Neurosci.* 1995;7:1603-1613.

513. Couratier P, Lesort M, Terro F, Dussartre C, Hugon J. NMDA antagonist blockade of AT8 tau immunoreactive changes in neuronal cultures. *Fundam Clin Pharmacol.* 1996;10:344-349.

514. Iqbal K, Li L, Sengupta A, Grundke-Iqbal I. Memantine restores okadaic acid-induced changes in protein phosphatase-2A, CAMKII and tau hyperphosphorylation in rat. *J Neurochem.* 2003;85:S43.

515. Wenk GL, Danysz W, Mobley SL. Investigations of neurotoxicity and neuroprotection within the nucleus basalis of the rat. *Brain Res.* 1994;655:7-11.

516. Wenk GL, Danysz W, Mobley SL. MK-801, memantine and amantadine show neuroprotective activity in the nucleus basalis magnocellularis. *Eur J Pharmacol.* 1995;293:267-270.

517. Welsh KA, Fillenbaum G, Wilkinson W, et al. Neuropsychological test performance in African-American and white patients with Alzheimer's Disease. *Neurology.* 1995;45:2207-2211.

518. Winblad B, Poritis N. Memantine in severe dementia: results of the 9M-Best Study (benefit and efficacy in severely demented patients during treatment with memantine). *Int J Geriatr Psychiatry.* 1999;14:135-146.

519. Reisberg B, Doody R, Stoffler A, Schmitt F, Ferris S, Mobius HF; Memantine Study Group. Memantine in moderate-to-severe Alzheimer's disease. *N Engl J Med.* 2003;348:1333-1341.

520. Tariot PN, Farlow MR, Grossberg GT, Graham SM, McDonald S, Gergel I; Memantine Study Group. Memantine treatment in patients with moderate to severe Alzheimer disease already receiving donepezil: a randomized controlled trial. *JAMA.* 2004;291:317-324.

521. Oreland L, Gottfries CG. Brain and brain monoamine oxidase in aging and in dementia of Alzheimer's type. *Prog Neuropsychopharmacol Biol Psychiatry.* 1986;10:533-540.

522. Smith CD, Carney JM, Starke-Reed PE, et al. Excess brain protein oxidation and enzyme dysfunction in normal aging and Alzheimer disease. *Proc Natl Acad Sci USA.* 1991;88:10540-10543.

523. Behl C, Davis J, Cole GM, Schubert D. Vitamin E protects nerve cells from amyloid beta protein toxicity. *Biochem Biophys Res Commun.* 1992;186:944-950.

12

524. Breitner JCS, Anthony JC, Khachaturian AS, Stone SV, Zaindi PP. Reduced risk of Alzheimer's disease in users of antioxidant vitamin supplements. The Cache County Study. *Neurobiol Aging*. 2002;23: S273.

525. Corrada MM, Breitner JCS, Brookmeyer R, Hallfrisch J, Muller DC, Kawas CH. Reduced risk of Alzheimer's disease with antioxidant vitamin intake: The Baltimore Longitudinal Study of Aging. *Neurobiol Aging*. 2002;23:S272.

526. Zandi PP, Anthony JC, Khachaturian AS, et al; Cache County Study Group. Reduced risk of Alzheimer disease in users of antioxidant vitamin supplements: the Cache County Study. *Arch Neurol*. 2004;61:82-88.

527. Luchsinger JA, Tang MX, Shea S, Mayeux R. Antioxidant vitamin intake and risk of Alzheimer disease. *Arch Neurol*. 2003;60:203-208.

528. Laurin D, Masaki KH, Foley DJ, White LR, Launer LJ. Midlife dietary intake of antioxidants and risk of late-life incident dementia: the Honolulu-Asia Aging Study. *Am J Epidemiol*. 2004;159:959-967.

529. Foley DJ, White LR. Dietary intake of antioxidants and risk of Alzheimer disease: food for thought. *JAMA*. 2002;287:3261-3263.

530. Corey-Bloom J, Thal LJ. Monoamine oxidase inhibitors in Alzheimer's disease. In: Lieberman A, Olanow CW, Youdim MBH, Tipton K, eds. *Monoamine Oxidase Inhibitors in Alzheimer's Disease*. New York, NY: Chapman and Hall Medical; 1994:279-294.

531. Sano M, Ernesto C, Thomas RG, et al. A controlled trial of selegiline, alpha-tocopherol, or both as treatment for Alzheimer's disease. The Alzheimer's Disease Cooperative Study. *N Engl J Med*. 1997;336: 1216-1222.

532. Gillis JC, Benefield P, McTavish D. Idebenone. A review of its pharmacodynamic and pharmacokinetic properties, and therapeutic use in age-related cognitive disorders. *Drugs Aging*. 1994;5:133-152.

533. Senin U, Parnetti L, Barbagallo-Sangiorgi G, et al. Idebenone in senile dementia of Alzheimer type: a multicentre study. *Arch Gerontol Geriatr*. 1992;15:249-260.

534. Bergamasco B, Scarzella L, La Commare P. Idebenone, a new drug in the treatment of cognitive impairment in patients with dementia of the Alzheimer type. *Funct Neurol*. 1994;9:161-168.

535. Weyer G, Babej-Dolle RM, Hadler D, Hofmann S, Herrmann WM. A controlled study of 2 doses of idebenone in the treatment of Alzheimer's disease. *Neuropsychobiology*. 1997;36:73-82.

536. Thal LJ, Grundman M, Berg J, et al. Idebenone treatment fails to slow cognitive decline in Alzheimer's disease. *Neurology*. 2003;61:1498-1502.

537. Packer L, Haramaki N, Kawabata T, et al. Ginkgo biloba extract (EGb 761). In: Christen Y, Courtois Y, Droy-Lefaix MT, et al, eds. *Ginkgo Biloba Extract (EGb 761) on Aging and Age-Related Disorders*. New York, NY: Elsevier Science; 1995.

538. Hofferberth B. The efficacy of EGb 761 in patients with senile dementia of the Alzheimer type: a double-blind placebo-controlled study on different levels of investigation. *Human Psychopharm*. 1994;9:215-222.

539. Maurer K, Ihl R, Dierks T, Frolich L. Clinical efficacy of Ginkgo biloba special extract EGb 761 in dementia of the Alzheimer type. *J Psychiatr Res*. 1997;31:645-655.

540. Le Bars PL, Katz MM, Berman N, Itil TM, Freedman AM, Schatzberg AF. A placebo-controlled, double-blind, randomized trial of an extract of Ginkgo biloba for dementia. North American EGb Study Group. *JAMA*. 1997;278:1327-1332.

541. Kanowski S, Hoerr R. Ginkgo biloba extract EGb 761 in dementia: intent-to-treat analyses of a 24-week, multi-center, double-blind, placebo controlled, randomized trial. *Pharmacopsychiatry*. 2003;36:297-303.

542. van Dongen M, van Rossum E, Kessels A, Sielhorst H, Knipschild P. Ginkgo for elderly people with dementia and age-associated memory impairment: a randomized clinical trial. *J Clin Epidemiol*. 2003;56:367-376.

543. Morris MC, Evans DA, Bienias JL, et al. Consumption of fish and n-3 fatty acids and risk of incident Alzheimer disease. *Arch Neurol*. 2003;60:940-946.

544. Aisen PS, Davis KL. Inflammatory mechanisms in Alzhheimer's disease: implications for therapy. *Am J Psychiatry*. 1994;151:1105-1113.

545. Breitner JC, Welsh KA, Helms MJ, et al. Delayed onset of Alzheimer's disease with nonsteroidal anti-inflammatory and histamine H2 blocking drugs. *Neurobiol Aging*. 1995;16:523-530.

546. McGeer PL, Schulzer M, McGeer EG. Arthritis and anti-inflammatory agents as possible protective factors for Alzheimer's disease: a review of 17 epidemiologic studies. *Neurology*. 1996;47:425-432.

547. Stewart WF, Kawas C, Corrada M, Metter EJ. Risk of Alzheimer's disease and duration of NSAID use. *Neurology*. 1997;48:626-632.

548. in t'Veld BA, Ruitenberg A, Hofman A, et al. Nonsteroidal antiinflammatory drugs and the risk of Alzheimer's disease. *N Engl J Med*. 2001;345:1515-1521.

549. Zandi PP, Anthony JC, Hayden KM, Mehta K, Mayer L, Breitner JC; Cache County Study Investigators. Reduced incidence of AD with NSAID but not H2 receptor antagonists: the Cache County Study. *Neurology*. 2002;59:880-886.

550. Wolfson D, Perrault A, Moride Y, Esdaile JM, Abenhaim L, Momoli F. A case-control analysis of nonsteroidal anti-inflammatory drugs and Alzheier's disease: are they protective. *Neuroepidmiology*. 2002;21:81-86.

551. Szekely CA, Thorne JE, Zandi PP, et al. Nonsteroidal anti-inflammatory drugs for the prevention of Alzheimer's disease: A systematic review. 2004. In press.

552. Aisen PS, Marin D, Alsteil L, et al. A pilot study of prednisone in Alzheimer's disease. *Dementia*. 1996;7:201-206.

553. Rogers J, Kirby LC, Hempelman SR, et al. Clinical trial of indomethacin in Alzheimer's disease. *Neurology*. 1993;43:1609-1611.

554. Vane J. Towards a better aspirin. *Nature*. 1994;367:215-216.

555. Aisen PS, Schmeidler J, Pasinetti GM. Randomized pilot study of nimesulide treatment in Alzheimer's disease. *Neurology*. 2002;58: 1050-1054.

556. Aisen PS, Davis KL, Berg JD, et al. A randomized controlled trial of prednisone in Alzheimer's disease. Alzheimer's Disease Cooperative Study. *Neurology*. 2000;54:588-593.

557. Aisen PS, Schafer KA, Grundman M, et al; Alzheimer's Disease Cooperative Study. Effects of rofecoxib or naproxen vs placebo on Alzheimer disease progression: a randomized controlled trial. *JAMA*. 2003;289:2819-2826.

12

558. Reines SA, Block GA, Morris JC, et al; Rofecoxib Protocol 091 Study Group. Rofecoxib: no effect on Alzheimer's disease in a 1-year, randomized, blinded, controlled study. *Neurology.* 2004;62:66-71.

559. Visser H, Thal L, Ferris S, et al. A randomized, double-blind, placebo-controlled study of rofecoxib in patients with mild cognitive impairment. 42nd Annual Meeting of the American College of Neuropsychopharmacology. San Juan, Puerto Rico.

560. Martin BK, Meinert CL, Breitner JC; ADAPT Research Group. Double placebo design in a prevention trial for Alzheimer's disease. *Control Clin Trials.* 2002;23:93-99.

561. Birge SJ. The role of estrogen in the treatment of Alzheimer's disease. *Neurology.* 1997;48(suppl 5):S36-S41.

562. Toran-Allerand CD, Miranda RC, Bentham WDL, et al. Estrogen receptors colocalize with low-affinity nerve growth factor receptors in cholinergic neurons of the basal forebrain. *Proc Natl Acad Sci USA.* 1992;89:4668-4672.

563. Woolley CS, McEwen BS. Estradiol regulates hippocampal dendritic spine density via an N-methyl-D-aspartate receptor-dependent mechanism. *J Neurosci.* 1994;14:7680-7687.

564. deLignieres B, Vincens M. Differential effects of exogenous oestradiol and progesterone on mood in postmenopausal women: individual dose effect relationship. *Maturitas.* 1982;4:67-72.

565. Yaffe K, Grady D, Pressman A, Cummings S. Serum estrogen levels, cognitive performance, and risk of cognitive decline in older community women. *J Am Geriatr Soc.* 1998;46:816-821.

566. Kawas C, Resnick S, Morrison A, et al. A prospective study of estrogen replacement therapy and the risk of developing Alzheimer's disease: the Baltimore Longitudinal Study of Aging [published correction appears in *Neurology.* 1998;51:654]. *Neurology.* 1997;48: 1517-1521.

567. Tang MX, Jacobs D, Stern Y, et al. Effect of oestrogen during menopause on risk and age at onset of Alzheimer's disease. *Lancet.* 1996;348:429-432.

568. Zandi PP, Carlson MC, Plassman BL, et al; Cache County Memory Study Investigators. Hormone replacement therapy and incidence of Alzheimer disease in older women: the Cache County Study. *JAMA.* 2002;288:2123-2129.

569. Henderson VW, Benke K, Green RC, Cupples LA, Farrer LA. Postmenopausal hormone therapy and Alzheimer's disease risk: Interaction with age. *J Neurol Neurosurg Psychiatr.* 2004. In press.

570. Barrett-Connor E. Rethinking estrogen and the brain. *JAGS.* 1998;46:918-920.

571. Barrett-Connor E, Grady D. Hormone replacement therapy, heart disease, and other considerations. *Annu Rev Pub Hlth.* 1998;19:55-72.

572. Espeland MA, Rapp SR, Shumaker SA, et al. Conjugated equine estrogens and global cognitive function in postmenopausal women: Women's Health Initiative Memory Study. *JAMA.* 2004;291:2959-2968.

573. Shumaker SA, Legault C, Rapp SR, et al; WHIMS Investigators. Estrogen plus progestin and the incidence of dementia and mild cognitive impairment in postmenopausal women: the Women's Health Initiative Memory Study: a randomized controlled trial. *JAMA.* 2003;289:2651-2662.

574. Shumaker SA, Legault C, Kuller L, et al. Conjugated equine estrogens and incidence of probable dementia and mild cognitive impairment in postmenopausal women. *JAMA.* 2004;2912947-2958.

575. Mulnard RA, Cotman CW, Kawas C, et al. Estrogen replacement therapy for treatment of mild to moderate Alzheimer disease: a randomized controlled trial. Alzheimer's Disease Cooperative Study. *JAMA.* 2000;283:1007-1015.

576. Henderson VW, Paganini-Hill A, Miller BL, et al. Estrogen for Alzheimer's disease in women: randomized, double-blind, placebo-controlled trial. *Neurology.* 2000;54:295-301.

577. Wolkowitz OM, Kramer JH, Reus VI, et al; DHEA-Alzheimer's Disease Collaborative Research. DHEA treatment of Alzheimer's disease: a randomized, double-blind, placebo-controlled study. *Neurology.* 2003;60:1071-1076.

578. Patel SV. Pharmacotherapy of cognitive impairment in Alzheimer's disease: a review. *J Geriatr Psychiatry Neurol.* 1995;8:81-95.

579. Jaffe J, Martin W. Opioid analgesics and antagonists. In: Gilman A, Goodman L, Gilman A, eds. *Pharmacological Basis of Therapeutics.* 6th ed. New York, NY: McMillan, 1980:494.

580. Arnsten AFT. Behavioral effects of naloxone in animals and humans: potential for treatment of aging disorders. In: Wurtman RJ, Corkin SH, Growdon JH, eds. *Alzheimer's Disease: Advances in Basic Research and Therapies. Proceedings of the Third Meeting of the International Study Group on Treatment of Memory Disorders Associated with Aging.* Zurich, Switzerland: Center for Brain Sciences and Metabolism Charitable Trust; 1984:407.

581. Blass J, Reding MJ, Drachman D, et al. Cholinesterase inhibitors and opiate antagonists in patients with Alzheimer's disease. *N Engl J Med.* 1983;309:556.

582. Henderson VW, Roberts E, Wimer C, et al. Multicenter trial of naloxone in Alzheimer's disease. *Ann Neurol.* 1989;25:404-406.

583. Flicker C, Ferris SH, Kalkstein D, Serby M. A double-blind, placebo-controlled crossover study of ganglioside GM_1 treatment for Alzheimer's disease. *Am J Psychiatry.* 1994;151:126-129.

584. Mohr E, Schlegel J, Fabbrini G, et al. Clonidine treatment of Alzheimer's disease. *Arch Neurol.* 1989;46:376-378.

585. Schlegel J, Mohr E, Williams J, Mann U, Gearing M, Chase TN. Guanfacine treatment of Alzheimer's disease. *Clin Neuropharmacol.* 1989;12:124-128.

586. Mouradian MM, Blin J, Giuffra M, et al. Somatostatin replacement therapy for Alzheimer dementia. *Ann Neurol.* 1991;30:610-613.

587. Nolan KA, Black RS, Sheu KF, Langberg J, Blass JP. A trial of thiamine in Alzheimer's disease. *Arch Neurol.* 1991;48:81-83.

588. Newhouse PA, Sunderland T, Tariot PN, et al. Intravenous nicotine in Alzheimer's disease: a pilot study. *Psychopharmacology.* 1988;95:171-175.

589. Jones GM, Sahakian BJ, Levy R, Warburton DM, Gray JA. Effects of acute subcutaneous nicotine on attention, information processing and short-term memory in Alzheimer's disease. *Psychopharmacology.* 1992;108:485-494.

590. Ban TA, Morey L, Aguglia E, et al. Nimodipine in the treatment of old age dementias. *Prog Neuropsychopharmacol Biol Psychiatry.* 1990;14:525-551.

12

591. Spagnoli A, Lucca U, Menasce G, et al. Long-term acetyl-L-carnitine treatment in Alzheimer's disease. *Neurology.* 1991;41:1726-1732.

592. Pettegrew JW, Klunk WE, Panchalingam K, Kanfer JN, McClure RJ. Clinical and neurochemical effects of acetyl-L-carnitine in Alzheimer's disease. *Neurobiol Aging.* 1995;16:1-4.

593. Manning CA, Ragozzino ME, Gold PE. Glucose enhancement of memory in patients with probable senile dementia of the Alzheimer's type. *Neurobiol Aging.* 1993;14:523-528.

594. Olson L. NGF and the treatment of Alzheimer's disease. *Exp Neurol.* 1993;124:5-15.

595. Grundman M, Capparelli E, Kim HT, et al; Alzheimer's Disease Co-operative Study. A multicenter, randomized, placebo controlled, multiple-dose safety and pharmacokinetic study of AIT-082 (Neotrofin) in mild Alzheimer's disease patients. *Life Sci.* 2003;73:539-553.

596. Claus JJ, Ludwig C, Mohr E, Giuffra M, Blin J, Chase TN. Nootropic drugs in Alzheimer's disease: symptomatic treatment with pramiracetam. *Neurology.* 1991;41:570-574.

597. Green RC, Goldstein FC, Auchus AP, et al. Treatment trial of oxiractam in Alzheimer's disease. *Arch Neurol.* 1992;49:1135-1136.

598. Mondadori C. Nootropics: preclinical results in the light of clinical effects; comparison with tacrine. *Crit Rev Neurobiol.* 1996;10:357-370.

599. Ruther E, Ritter R, Apecechea M, Freytag S, Windisch M. Efficacy of the peptidergic nootropic drug cerebrolysin in patients with senile dementia of the Alzheimer type (SDAT). *Pharmacopsychiatry.* 1994;27:32-40.

600. Ruther E, Ritter R, Apecechea M, Freytag S, Gmeinbauer R, Windisch M. Sustained improvements in patients with dementia of Alzheimer's type (DAT) 6 months after termination of Cerebroylsin therapy. *J Neural Transm.* 2000;107:815-829.

601. Panisset M, Gauthier S, Moessler H, Windisch M; Cerebrolysin Study Group. Cerebrolysin in Alzheimer's disease: a randomized, double-blind, placebo-controlled trial with a neurotrophic agent. *J Neural Transm.* 2002;109:1089-1104.

602. Schenk D, Barbour R, Dunn W, et al. Immunization with amyloid-beta attenuates Alzheimer-disease-like pathology in the PDAPP mouse. *Nature.* 1999;400:173-177.

603. Bard F, Cannon C, Barbour R, et al. Peripherally administered antibodies against amyloid beta-peptide enter the central nervous system and reduce pathology in a mouse model of Alzheimer disease. *Nat Med.* 2000;6:916-919.

604. Janus C, Pearson J, McLaurin J, et al. A beta peptide immunization reduces behavioural impairment and plaques in a model of Alzheimer's disease. *Nature.* 2000;408:979-982.

605. Orgogozo JM, Gilman S, Dartigues JF, et al. Subacute meningoencephalitis in a subset of patients with AD after Abeta42 immunization. *Neurology.* 2003;61:46-54.

606. Munch G, Robinson SR. Potential neurotoxic inflammatory responses to Abeta vaccination in humans. *J Neural Transm.* 2002;109:1081-1087.

607. Nath A, Hall E, Tuzova M, et al. Autoantibodies to amyloid beta-peptide (Abeta) are increased in Alzheimer's disease patients and Abeta antibodies can enhance Abeta neurotoxicity: implications for disease

pathogenesis and vaccine development. *Neuromolecular Med.* 2003;3:29-39.

608. Nicoll JA, Wilkinson D, Holmes C, Steart P, Markham H, Weller RO. Neuropathology of human Alzheimer disease after immunization with amyloid-beta peptide: a case report. *Nat Med.* 2003;9:448-452.

609. Hock C, Konietzko U, Streffer JR, et al. Antibodies against beta-amyloid slow cognitive decline in Alzheimer's disease. *Neuron.* 2003;38:547-554.

610. Robinson SR, Bishop GM, Munch G. Alzheimer vaccine: amyloid-beta on trial. *Bioessays.* 2003;25:283-288.

611. Michaelis ML, Dobrowsky RT, Li G. Tau neurofibrillary pathology and microtubule stability. *J Mol Neurosci.* 2002;19:289-293.

612. Roder HM. Prospect of therapeutic approaches to tauopathies. *J Mol Neurosci.* 2003;20:195-202.

613. Jick H, Zornberg GL, Jick SS, Seshadri S, Drachman DA. Statins and the risk of dementia. *Lancet.* 2000;356:1627-1631.

614. Wolozin B, Kellman W, Ruosseau P, Celesia GG, Siegel G. Decreased prevalence of Alzheimer disease associated with 3-hydroxy-3-methyglutaryl coenzyme A reductase inhibitors. *Arch Neurol.* 2000;57:1439-1443.

615. Rockwood K, Kirkland S, Hogan DB, et al. Use of lipid-lowering agents, indication bias, and the risk of dementia in community-dwelling elderly people. *Arch Neurol.* 2002;59:223-227.

616. Green RC, McNagny SE, Jayakumar P, Cupples LA, Benke K, Farrer LA. Statin use and the risk of Alzheimer's disease. *Neurology.* 2005. In submission.

617. Li G, Higdon R, Kukull WA, et al. Statin therapy and risk of dementia in the elderly: a community-based prospective cohort study. *Neurology.* 2004;63:1624-1628.

618. Zandi PP, Sparks DL, Khachaturian A, et al. Do statins reduce risk of incident dementia and AD? The Cache County Study. *Arch Gen Psychiatry.* 2004. In press.

619. Cherny RA, Atwood CS, Xilinas ME, et al. Treatment with a copper-zinc chelator markedly and rapidly inhibits beta-amyloid accumulation in Alzheimer's disease transgenic mice. *Neuron.* 2001;30:665-676.

620. Regland B, Lehmann W, Abedini I, et al. Treatment of Alzheimer's disease with clioquiniol. *Dement Geriatr Cogn Disord.* 2001;12:408-414.

621. Scarmeas N, Levy G, Tang MX, Manly J, Stern Y. Influence of leisure activity on the incidence of Alzheimer's disease. *Neurology.* 2001;57:2236-2242.

622. Wilson RS, Mendes De Leon CF, Barnes LL, et al. Participation in cognitively stimulating activities and risk of incident Alzheimer disease. *JAMA.* 2002;287:742-748.

623. Fillit HM, Butler RN, O'Connell AW, et al. Achieving and maintaining cognitive vitality with aging. *Mayo Clin Proc.* 2002;77:681-696.

624. Silverberg GD, Levinthal E, Sullivan EV, et al. Assessment of low-flow CSF drainage as a treatment for AD: results of a randomized pilot study. *Neurology.* 2002;59:1139-1145.

625. Goldsmith HS. Treatment of Alzheimer's disese by transposition of the omentum. *Ann NY Acad Sci.* 2002;977:454-467.

626. Goldsmith HS, Wu W, Zhong J, Edgar M. Omental transposition to the brain as a surgical method for treating Alzheimer's disease. *Neurol Res.* 2003;25:625-634.

12

627. Diamond B, Johnson S, Torsney K, et al. Complementary and alternative medicines in the treatment of dementia: an evidence-based review. *Drugs Aging.* 2003;20:981-998.

628. Hall GR. Care of the patient with Alzheimer's disease living at home. *Nurs Clin North Am.* 1988;23:31-46.

629. Chenoweth B, Spencer B. Dementia: the experience of family caregivers. *Gerontologist.* 1986;26:267-272.

630. Scarmeas N, Brandt J, Albert M, et al. Association between the APOE genotype and psychopathologic symptoms in Alzheimer's disease. *Neurology.* 2002;58:1182-1188.

631. Craig D, Hart DJ, McCool K, McIlroy SP, Passmore AP. Apolipoprotein E e4 allele influences aggressive behaviour in Alzheimer's disease. *J Neurol Neurosurg Psychiatry.* 2004;75:1327-1330.

632. Lyketsos CG, Lopez O, Jones B, Fitzpatrick AL, Breitner J, DeKosky S. Prevalence of neuropsychiatric symptoms in dementia and mild cognitive impairment: results from the cardiovascular health study. *JAMA.* 2002;288:1475-1483.

633. Chan DC, Kasper JD, Black BS, Rabins PV. Prevalence and correlates of behavioral and psychiatric symptoms in community-dwelling elders with dementia or mild cognitive impairment: the Memory and Medical Care Study. *Int J Geriatr Psychiatry.* 2003;18:174-182.

634. Holtzer R, Tang MX, Devanand DP, et al. Psychopathological features in Alzheimer's disease: course and relationship with cognitive status. *J Am Geriatr Soc.* 2003;51:953-960.

635. Tariot PN, Podgorski CA, Blazina L, Leibovici A. Mental disorders in the nursing home: another perspective. *Am J Psychiatry.* 1993;150:1063-1069.

636. Cohen-Mansfield J. Assessment of agitation. *Int Psychogeriatr.* 1996;8:233-245.

637. Murman DL, Chen Q, Powell MC, Kuo SB, Bradley CJ, Colenda CC. The incremental direct costs associated with behavioral symptoms in AD. *Neurology.* 2002;59:1721-1729.

638. Rabins PV. Noncognitive symptoms in Alzheimer disease. Definitions, treatments, and possible etiologies. In: Terry RD, Katzman R, Bick KL, eds. *Alzheimer Disease.* New York, NY: Raven Press; 1994.

639. Mega MS, Cummings JL, Fiorello T, Gornbein J. The spectrum of behavioral changes in Alzheimer's disease. *Neurology.* 1996;46:130-135.

640. Tariot PN. Treatment strategies for agitation and psychosis in dementia. *J Clin Psychiatry.* 1996;57(suppl):S21-S29.

641. Cummings JL. The neuropsychiatric inventory: assessing psychopathology in dementia patients. *Neurology.* 1997;48(suppl):S10-S16.

642. Devanand DP, Jacobs DM, Tang MX, et al. The course of psychopathologic features in mild to moderate Alzheimer disease. *Arch Gen Psychiatry.* 1997;54:257-263.

643. Volicer L, Hurley AC. Management of behavioral symptoms in progressive degenerative dementias. *J Gerontol A Biol Sci Med Sci.* 2003;58:M837-M845.

644. Bassiony MM, Lyketsos CG. Delusions and hallucinations in Alzheimer's disease: review of the brain decade. *Psychosomatics.* 2003;44:388-401.

645. Lachs MS, Becker M, Siegal AP, Miller RL, Tinetti ME. Delusions and behavioral disturbances in cognitively impaired elderly persons. *J Am Geriatr Soc.* 1992;40:768-773.

646. Cummings JL. Organic delusions: phenomenology, anatomical correlations, and review. *Br J Psychiatry.* 1985;146:184-197.

647. Logsdon RG, Teri L, McCurry SM, Gibbons LE, Kukull WA, Larson EB. Wandering: a significant problem among community-residing individuals with Alzheimer's disease. *J Gerontol B Psychol Sci Soc Sci.* 1998;53:P294-P299.

648. Mahoney EK, Volicer L, Hurley AC. *Management of Challenging Behaviors in Dementia.* Baltimore, Md: Health Professionals Press; 2000.

649. Algase DL, Beattie ER, Leitsch SA, Beel-Bates CA. Biomechanical activity devices to index wandering behavior in dementia. *Am J Alzheimers Dis Other Demen.* 2003;18:85-92.

650. Lyketsos CG, Olin J. Depression in Alzheimer's disease: overview and treatment. *Biol Psychiatry.* 2002;52:243-252.

651. Payne JL, Sheppard JM, Steinberg M, et al. Incidence, prevalence, and outcomes of depression in residents of a long-term care facility with dementia. *Int J Geriatr Psychiatry.* 2002;17:247-253.

652. Lyketsos CG, Lee HB. Diagnosis and treatment of depression in Alzheimer's disease. A practical update for the clinician. *Dement Geriatr Cogn Disord.* 2004;17:55-64.

653. Lyketsos CG, Tune LE, Pearlson G, Steele C. Major depression in Alzheimer's disease. An interaction between gender and family history. *Psychosomatics.* 1996;37:380-384.

654. Strauss ME, Ogrocki PK. Confirmation of an association between family history of affective disorder and the depressive syndrome in Alzheimer's disease. *Am J Psychiatry.* 1996;153:1340-1342.

655. Lyketsos CG, DelCampo L, Steinberg M, et al. Treating depression in Alzheimer disease: efficacy and safety of sertraline therapy, and the benefits of depression reduction: the DIADS. *Arch Gen Psychiatry.* 2003;60:737-746.

656. Rabins PV, Mace NL, Lucas MJ. The impact of dementia on the family. *JAMA.* 1982;248:333-335.

657. Gierz M, Campbell SS, Gillin JC. Sleep disturbances in various nonaffective psychiatric disorders. *Psychiatr Clin North Am.* 1987;10:565-581.

658. Sanford JRA. Tolerance of debility in elderly dependents by supporters at home: its significance for hospital practice. *BMJ.* 1975;3:471-473.

659. Ancoli-Israel S, Parker L, Sinaee R, Fell RL, Kripke DF. Sleep fragmentation in patients from a nursing home. *J Gerontol.* 1989;44:M18-M21.

660. Jacobs D, Ancoli-Israel S, Parker L, Kripke DF. Twenty-four-hour sleep-wake patterns in a nursing home population. *Psychol Aging.* 1989;4:352-356.

661. Reynolds CF 3d, Hoch CC, Stack J, Campbell D. The nature and management of sleep/wake disturbance in Alzheimer's dementia. *Psychopharmacol Bull.* 1988;24:43-48.

662. Cohen-Mansfield J, Watson V, Meade W, Gordon M, Leatherman J, Emor C. Does sundowning occur in residents of an Alzheimer's unit. *Int J Geriatr Psychiatry.* 1989;4:293-298.

663. Riviere S, Gillette-Guyonnet S, Andrieu S, et al. Cognitive function and caregiver burden: predictive factors for eating behaviour disorders in Alzheimer's disease. *Int J Geriatr Psychiatry.* 2002;17:950-955.

12

664. Volicer L. Clinical guidelines for the treatment of Alzheimer's disease and other progressive dementias. *Fed Pract Suppl.* 1999;May:16-25.

665. Teri L, Gibbons LE, McCurry SM, et al. Exercise plus behavioral management in patients with Alzheimer disease: a randomized controlled trial. *JAMA.* 2003;290:2015-2022.

666. Zeisel J, Silverstein NM, Hyde J, Levkoff S, Lawton MP, Holmes W. Environmental correlates to behavioral health outcomes in Alzheimer's special care units. *Gerontologist.* 2003;43:697-711.

667. Teri L, Logsdon RG, McCurry SM. Nonpharmacologic treatment of behavioral disturbance in dementia. *Med Clin North Am.* 2002;86:641-656.

668. Gray KF. Managing agitation and difficult behavior in dementia. *Clin Geriatr Med.* 2004;20:69-82.

669. Volicer L, Hurley AC, Mahoney E. Management of behavioral symptoms of dementia. *Nursing Home Medicine.* 1995;3:300-306.

670. Mintzer JE, Hoernig KS, Mirski DF. Treatment of agitation in patients with dementia. *Clin Geriatr Med.* 1998:14:147-175.

671. Alexopoulos GS, Silver JM, Kahn DA, Frances A, Carpenter D. Treatment of agitation in older persons with dementia. *Expert Consensus Guideline Series: A Special Report of Postgraduate Medicine,* 1998.

672. Cummings JL. Alzheimer's disease. *N Engl J Med.* 2004;351:56-67.

673. Profenno LA, Tariot PN. Pharmacologic management of agitation in Alzheimer's disease. *Dement Geriatr Cogn Disord.* 2004;17:65-77.

674. Teri L, Logsdon RG, Peskind E, et al; Alzheimer's Disease Cooperative Study. Treatment of agitation in AD: a randomized, placebo-controlled clinical trial. *Neurology.* 2000;55:1271-1278.

675. Allain H, Dautzenberg PH, Maurer K, Schuck S, Bonhomme D, Gerard D. Double blind study of tiapride versus haloperidol and placebo in agitation and aggressiveness in elderly patients with cognitive impairment. *Psychopharmacology.* 2000;148:361-366.

676. Lanctot KL, Best TS, Mittmann N, et al. Efficacy and safety of neuroleptics in behavioral disorders associated with dementia. *J Clin Psychiatry.* 1998;59:550-561.

677. Lee PE, Gill SS, Freedman M, Bronskill SE, Hillmer MP, Rochon PA. Atypical antipsychotic drugs in the treatment of behavioural and psychological symptoms of dementia: systematic review. *BMJ.* 2004;329:75.

678. Volicer L, Rheaume Y, Cyr D. Treatment of depression in advanced Alzheimer's disease using sertraline. *J Geriatr Psychiatry Neurol.* 1994;7:227-229.

679. Tariot PN, Loy R, Ryan JM, Porsteinsson A, Ismail S. Mood stabilizers in Alzheimer's disease: symptomatic and neuroprotective rationales. *Adv Drug Deliv Rev.* 2002;54:1567-1577.

680. Tariot PN, Erb R, Podgorski CA, et al. Efficacy and tolerability of carbamazepine for agitation and aggression in dementia. *Am J Psychiatry.* 1998;155:54-61.

681. Porsteinsson AP, Tariot PN, Erb R, et al. Placebo-controlled study of divalproex sodium for agitation in dementia. *Am J Geriatr Psychiatry.* 2001;9:58-66.

682. Tariot PN, Schneider L, Mintzer J, et al. Safety and tolerability of divalproex sodium for the treatment of signs and symptoms of mania in elderly persons wtih dementia: Results of a double-blind, placebo-controlled trial. *Curr Therapeutic Res.* 2001;62:51-67.

683. Sival RC, Haffmans PM, Jansen PA, Duursma SA, Eikelenboom P. Sodium valproate in the treatment of aggressive behavior in patients with dementia—a randomized placebo controlled clinical trial. *Int J Geriatr Psychiatry.* 2002;17:579-585.

684. Cummings JL, Cyrus PA, Gulanski B. Metrifonate efficacy in the treatment of psychiatric and behavioral disturbances of Alzheimer's disease patients. *American Geriatrics Society/American Federation for Aging Research.* Seattle, Wash; 1998.

685. Kaufer D, Cummings JL, Christine D. Differential neuropsychiatric symptom responses to tacrine in Alzheimer's disease: relationship to dementia severity. *J Neuropsychiatry Clin Neurosci.* 1998;10:55-63.

686. Tariot PN, Solomon PR, Morris JC, Kershaw P, Lilienfeld S, Ding C. A 5-month, randomized, placebo-controlled trial of galantamine in AD. The Galantamine USA-10 Study Group. *Neurology.* 2000;54:2269-2276.

687. Tariot PN, Cummings JL, Katz IR, et al. A randomized, double-blind, placebo-controlled study of the efficacy and safety of donepezil in patients with Alzheimer's disease in the nursing home setting. *J Am Geriatr Soc.* 2001;49:1590-1599.

688. Gauthier S, Feldman H, Hecker J, et al. Efficacy of donepezil on behavioral symptoms in patients with moderate to severe Alzheimer's disease. *Int Psychogeriatr.* 2002;14:389-404.

689. Paleacu D, Mazeh D, Mirecki I, Even M, Barak Y. Donepezil for the treatment of behavioral symptoms in patients with Alzheimer's disease. *Clin Neuropharmacol.* 2002;25:313-317.

690. Manfredi PL, Breuer B, Wallenstein S, Stegmann M, Bottomley G, Libow L. Opioid treatment for agitation in patients with advanced dementia. *Int J Geriatr Psychiatry.* 2003;18:700-705.

691. Singer C, Tractenberg RE, Kaye J, et al; Alzheimer's Disease Cooperative Study. A multicenter, placebo-controlled trial of melatonin for sleep disturbance in Alzheimer's disease. *Sleep.* 2003;26:893-901.

692. Lindgren CL. A caregiver career. *Image J Nurs Sch.* 1993;25:214-219.

693. Gwyther LP. Social issues of the Alzheimer's patient and family. *Am J Med.* 1998;104:17S-21S; discussion, 39S-42S.

694. Schulz R, Beach SR. Caregiving as a risk factor for mortality: the Caregiver Health Effects Study. *JAMA.* 1999;282:2215-2219.

695. Covinsky KE, Newcomer R, Fox P, et al. Patient and caregiver characteristics associated with depression in caregivers of patients with dementia. *J Gen Intern Med.* 2003;18:1006-1014.

696. Dunkin JJ, Anderson-Hanley C. Dementia caregiver burden: a review of the literature and guidelines for assessment and intervention. *Neurology.* 1998;51(suppl 1):S53-S60; discussion S65-S67.

697. White-Means SI, Thornton MC. Ethnic differences in the production of informal home health care. *Gerontologist.* 1990;30:758-768.

698. American Psychiatric Association. APA practice guidelines for the treatment of patients with Alzheimer's disease and other dementias in late life. *Am J Psychiatry.* 1997;154(suppl):1-39.

699. Rebok GW, Keyl PM, Bylsma FW, Blaustein MJ, Tune L. The effects of Alzheimer disease on driving-related abilities. *Alzheimer Dis Assoc Disord.* 1994;8:228-240.

700. Fitten LJ, Perryman KM, Wilkinson CJ, et al. Alzheimer and vascular dementias and driving. A prospective road and laboratory study. *JAMA.* 1995;273:1360-1365.

701. Fox GK, Bowden SC, Bashford GM, Smith DS. Alzheimer's disease and driving: prediction and assessment of driving performance. *J Am Geriatr Soc.* 1997;45:949-953.

702. Wild K, Cotrell V. Identifying driving impairment in Alzheimer disease: a comparison of self and observer reports versus driving evaluation. *Alzheimer Dis Assoc Disord.* 2003;17:27-34.

703. Green RC, Kellerman AL. Grandfather's gun: when should we intervene? *J Am Geriatr Soc.* 1996;44:467-469.

704. Griffith HR, Belue K, Sicola A, et al. Impaired financial abilities in mild cognitive impairment: a direct assessment approach. *Neurology.* 2003;60:449-457.

705. Hirschman KB, James BD, Joyce CM, et al. Do Alzheimer's disease patients want to participate in an AD treatment decision and will their family let them? *Neurobiol Aging.* 2004;25:21.

706. Karlawish JH, Bonnie RJ, Appelbaum PS, et al. Addressing the ethical, legal, and social issues raised by voting by persons with dementia. *JAMA.* 2004;292:1345-1350.

707. Pfeiffer E. Institutional placement for patients with Alzheimer's disease. How to help families with a difficult decision. *Postgrad Med.* 1995;97:125-126, 129-132.

708. Berg L, Buckwalter KC, Chafetz PK, et al. Special care units for persons with dementia. *J Am Geriatr Soc.* 1991;39:1229-1236.

709. Holmes D, Teresi J, Monaco C. Special care units in nursing homes: prevalence in five states. *Gerontologist.* 1992;32:191-196.

710. Maslow K. Consumer education, research, regulatory, and reimbursement issues in special care units. *Alzheimer Dis Assoc Disord.* 1994;8(suppl 1):S429-S433.

711. Schulz R, Mendelsohn AB, Haley WE, et al; Resources for Enhancing Alzheimer's Caregiver Health Investigators. End-of-life care and the effects of bereavement on family caregivers of persons with dementia. *N Engl J Med.* 2003;349:1936-1942.

712. Hurley AC, Volicer L. Alzheimer Disease: "It's okay, Mama, if you want to go, it's okay". *JAMA.* 2002;288:2324-2331.

INDEX

Note: Page numbers followed by f indicate figures and t indicate tables.
CP-1 and CP-2 indicate unpaged color plates.

13

233

13

13

13

13

13

244

13

13

13

13

13

253

13